Old Age
Health Challenges
and
Solutions

What happens to your Skin, Gut, Eyes, Teeth, Blood, and Sexuality when you grow old. Know about Psychological, Gynecological, Sleep Disorders, Temperature Regulation Palliative Care and End-of-Life Care in the Elderly

Problems of the Elderly Book 2.

Sahasranam Kalpathy

<u>COPYRIGHT</u>

Copyright © 2023 by Sahasranam Kalpathy All rights reserved. No part of this book may be produced or stored in a retrieval system or transmitted in any form by any means, electronic, photocopying, recording, or otherwise, without express written permission of the author.

Disclaimer

All the facts in the books and the statistics given are taken from authentic sources. The diagrams in the book are the author's own and drawn by the author himself and not reproduced from any other source. However, the personal opinions expressed throughout the book are the author's own. The diagrams in the book are drawn by the author himself. **This is not a book which can be used as a substitute for the physician.**

I dedicate this book to my good friend
Dr. K. G. Alexander
Chairman and Medical Director, Baby Memorial Hospital,
Calicut
whose compassionate leadership has set a
benchmark in patient Care.

PREFACE

Don't let age change you, change the way you age.

My intention in bringing out this series on the Problems of the Elderly was to promote the knowledge as to what happens to us when we become old. Often, old age is thought to be a curse and the elderly considered a burden on their family and society. The contributions of the elderly individuals when they were young and active in the society may be forgotten and they may be considered *'excess luggage'* in some families and are relegated to 'Old Age Homes' euphemistically called "Retirement Homes".

The elderly are entitled to their dignity and independence. But unfortunately, old age brings with it infirmities due to co-existing diseases which makes their life distressing, often needing dependence on a relative or a caregiver.

To know the abnormalities occurring in old age, one should understand normal aging. We should know what changes befall us normally with increasing age before we learn the diseases that assail us. This book ventures to give an insight into the 'normal' changes which one should expect when one crosses into the sunset years of life. Many of the 'normal' changes occurring in old age are symptomless, like cervical spondylosis and benign enlargement of the prostate. It is important to understand that such disease entities need no treatment if the patient is not troubled by these. Hence, a knowledge of these ailments becomes imperative. That is what this book aims to explain.

Many of the diseases of old age can be prevented if one is prudent in the early years of life following a healthy lifestyle and taking adequate health precautions. This book ventures to explain in simple terms some of the diseases encountered in the elderly, their causes, risk factors, symptoms, diagnostic methods, and a very brief account of how they are treated.

The main emphasis however has been on the ***Prevention*** of the diseases in the elderly, giving enough forethought to implement preventive strategies when one is young. This gives the elderly individuals a disease-free, disability-free life in their final years. One must remember that "*Aging is a privilege denied to many*".

This is **not** a book which can be used as a substitute for the physician. It is a book written for the common man to make one aware of the vagaries of old age. It is a book which helps the caregiver to understand the elderly individual's problems and concerns with empathy and respond to them benevolently.

Medical terminology has been used to a minimum and wherever they have been used, they have been explained in detail. Difficult medical words have been *italicized* and their definitions given in the **Glossary** at the end of the book.

Those readers who have not read the Book 1 of this series titled, ***"How to Face the Health Challenges while Growing Old"*** are encouraged to do so as these books together comprise a comprehensive health guide about old age afflictions.

The readers are kindly requested to give a review of the book after reading it. I hope the readers will benefit from my modest venture. With these words, I humbly present this book to my readers as a New Year gift in 2023.

Sahasranam Kalpathy

(Dr. K. V. Sahasranam MD. DM. FACC. FICS.)

INTRODUCTION

God ! grant me the serenity
To accept the things I cannot change,
Courage to change the things I can,
And
Wisdom to know the difference.

Old age is an inescapable milestone in human life. Over the past few decades, improvements in public health measures, sanitation, better health care, development of newer antibiotics and other medications, discovery of vaccinations for newer diseases and giant strides in the treatment of diseases have prolonged life and increased the lifespan of the average human being. Science and Technology has contributed in a great way to this revolution in medical care.

It is predicted that by the year 2045, elderly people over the age of 60 will exceed the number of children below 15 years of age. This reversal will be as a result of social, economic, and health development globally. This of course, will bring an additional economic burden on society and governments, to take care of the elderly who will seldom be productive members of society, but will draw upon the health and economic resources of the society and the government. This will pose a challenge to governments world over.

Many diseases of the elderly were discussed at length in Book 1 of this series called *"Problems of the Elderly"*. The book was titled *"How to Face the Health Challenges While Growing Old"*. This book presents additional insights into diseases not covered in the previous book of this series.

An elaborate account of diseases of the *Gastrointestinal system*, *Skin* and *Eye* are discussed in the first three chapters. This is followed by a discussion of the diseases of the *Blood*, the *Female Reproductive system*, and *Dental problems.*

Psychological diseases and *Sexuality* in the elderly have been discussed in detail. *Sleep disorders* and *Temperature regulation* which are an important aspect of the elderly individual's concern have been given due importance.

A chapter on *Miscellaneous disorders* has been included separately. *Cervical Spondylosis, Benign Hypertrophy of the Prostate, Hernia, Hemorrhoids, Back pain, and Frailty* which are common problems in both elderly males and females have been discussed. Emphasis on prevention has been given special consideration in the section on *Back Pain*.

The concluding chapter is on *Palliative care and End-of-Life Care*. As Death is an essential part of living, a section on *Living Will and Advance Medical Directive* has been added to familiarize the reader with this aspect of Elderly Care, especially since this is not mandatory in certain countries like India. The Living Will gives a person the privilege to die with dignity.

A **Glossary** at the end of the book acquaints the reader with some of the technical and medical terms used in the book. Difficult medical terms have been avoided and substituted by simple, easily understandable terms.

Each chapter describing diseases of the systems like Gastrointestinal system. Skin, Eye, Gynecological diseases, Dental problems, and Blood disorders are prefixed with a short Anatomical and Physiological description of the involved system. This is to familiarize the reader with the basic anatomy of the system, to help him understand the description of the diseases easily. This description of the anatomy is optional as the diseases are explained in simple English to be easily comprehended by the reader.

Black & white diagrams of the systems have been included in the chapters. The diagrams are drawn by the author himself and are a rough guide to understand the Anatomy of the systems. Pictorial accuracy cannot be guaranteed as the diagrams are hand-drawn.

1. THE GASTROINTESTINAL SYSTEM

Structure and Function. The Digestive System, or the Gastrointestinal System(**GIS**) extends from the mouth above to the anus below. It includes the stomach, the intestines, liver, pancreas, and the gall bladder. The main function of the GIS is to convert the food that we eat into nutrients and other substances that provide energy for the functioning of the body. These nutrients are absorbed into the blood and distributed to various parts of the body.

Mouth & Esophagus: The mouth is the first part of the GIS. Chewing the food breaks it into smaller particles that are easily digested. The saliva present in the mouth contains *enzymes* that partially digest the *carbohydrates* in the food. The esophagus (gullet) is the tube that conveys the swallowed food into the stomach. It has no digestive function.

Stomach: The esophagus leads to the stomach where digestion begins. The inner lining of the stomach secretes enzymes and acid. The acid is hydrochloric acid and it helps to break down the *proteins* and kill any bacteria present in food. The enzymes secreted by the stomach digest the proteins and carbohydrates. Certain nutrients are absorbed in the stomach. The stomach churns the food into smaller particles which can be easily digested when they reach the intestines.

The food in the GIS is propelled forward by a process called *Peristalsis*. The esophagus, stomach and intestines contain muscles in its wall. They contract and relax in a wave like fashion to propel the food forward like toothpaste being squeezed out of a tube. Peristalsis also helps the food to be intimately mixed with the juices in the stomach and intestines to help digestion. From the stomach, the food is passed into the small intestines for further digestion.

Small intestine. The small intestine is composed of three parts – Duodenum, Jejunum, and Ileum. It is called "small" because of its smaller diameter compared to the large intestines. The duodenum is the first part of the small intestines. The small intestine is the longest part of the gastrointestinal tract and is approximately 22 feet long. (**Figure 1**).

The Duodenum is the first part of the small intestine. It is "C" shaped and is 10 inches long. It continues as the Jejunum below. The duodenum receives the ducts from the pancreas and the liver. The food reaching the duodenum from the stomach mixes with the juices from the liver and pancreas and is passed on to the Jejunum below.

The Jejunum is the next part of the small intestine. It is about 8 feet long. The food in the jejunum is in a semisolid state and is churned to and fro by the contractions of the muscles in the wall of the small intestine. The digested food and water is absorbed here to some extent. The juices in the small intestine contain enzymes that further breakdown the proteins, fats, and carbohydrates in conjunction with the bile and the pancreatic juice.

The Ileum forms the rest of the small intestine. It continues the digestive process, churns the food, and absorbs nutrients and water. Maximum absorption of nutrients and water happens in the ileum. The food is then propelled forward by peristalsis into the large intestines.

The whole of the inner lining of the small intestine has many folds which increase the surface area so that a large area is available for digested nutrients to be absorbed. In addition, the intestinal lining has many tiny finger-like projections about ½ inch long called *Villi*. These intestinal villi further increase the area available for absorption. Hence most of the absorption of water and nutrients occurs in the small intestines. Blood vessels which are present in the wall of the intestine carry the absorbed nutrients to various parts of the body.

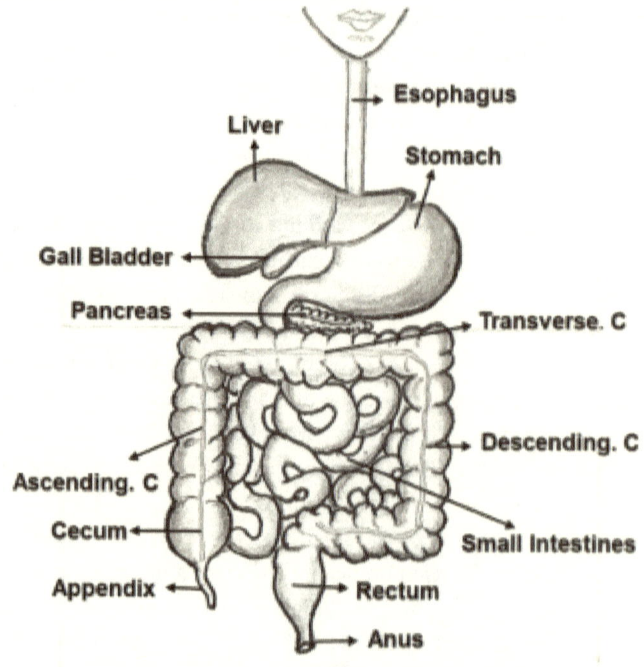

Figure 1

The Liver & Pancreas. The liver is an organ with many *metabolic* functions. One of the functions of the liver is to secrete Bile, a greenish-yellow juice which is stored in a sac – the Gall Bladder, situated below the liver. The bile is secreted into the duodenum through the bile *duct* when food reaches the duodenum. The bile helps to digest fat by breaking down the large fat globules into tiny particles (*Emulsification*). These tiny fat particles are then easily digested by the pancreatic and intestinal enzymes.

The Pancreas is a bitter-gourd shaped organ situated in the curvature of the duodenum. It secretes pancreatic juice which reaches the duodenum through the pancreatic *duct*. The pancreatic juice contains enzymes which digest proteins, fats, and carbohydrates.

Large Intestine. This is the continuation of the small intestine and has three parts, the *Colon, Rectum,* and *Anus.* The main function of the large intestine is the final absorption of water from the digested matter and converting it into *feces (stools)* which is excreted through the anus. The large intestines is about 5 feet long.

The large intestine has many parts. The part where the small intestine joins the large intestine is called the *Cecum.* It is pouch-like and is about 4-6 inches long. It is situated on the right lower part of the abdomen. A small worm like structure called the *Appendix* hangs down from the cecum. The main function of the cecum is to absorb water and minerals from the food residue.

Following the cecum are the three parts called the *Ascending,* (one the right side) *Transverse* (across the upper part of the abdomen) and *Descending* colon, (on the left side) so named because of their location. The descending colon continues to become an "S" – shaped tube called the *Sigmoid Colon.* It is situated in the left lower part of the abdomen and is about 10-15 inches long. Nutrients and water are absorbed from the large intestine.

The *Rectum* is the final part of the large intestine and connects the sigmoid colon to the anus. It is about 6-8 inches long. It stores the residual stools that enters it. When the individual decides to pass stools, the muscles in the rectum contract causing the stools to be evacuated through the anus.

The Anus or the Anal Canal is the last part of the GIS and is about 2 inches long. It has two strong muscle bands that form rings around it to prevent feces from being passed out involuntarily. These ring like muscles are called *Sphincters.*

When the feces fill the rectum, the person feels the urge to pass stools. When he sits on the toilet seat to pass stools, the sphincter muscles in the anus relax and the stool is passed out.

It is expected that 17% of the population in the world would be above the age of 80 by 2050. In the United States 14.5% of the population are above the age of 65 presently. As age advances, as in the other systems, changes occur in the Gastrointestinal system (**GIS**) also. As most of the medications that we consume are taken orally and are absorbed by the gut, side effects of these are seen often in the GIS. Maintaining good dietary habits is important in preserving the health of the gut in old age.

Changes in the mouth in old age are seen as a decrease in the quantity and quality of the saliva produced. Drying of mouth and taste disturbances often occur in old age.

In the esophagus, increasing age produces changes during swallowing and difficulties associated with it. Pain during swallowing, delayed swallowing, reflux disease, and *inflammation* of the esophagus due to medications may occur.

The stomach normally is lined by cells which can repair themselves whenever they are injured by any adverse factors. In the elderly, this repair function is impaired leading to stomach ulcer and peptic ulcer disease. Diseases like diabetes and Parkinson's disease, delay the emptying of the stomach and hence the food remains in the stomach for longer periods. The stomach is the commonest organ of the GIS which is easily affected by the side effects of medications in the elderly.

Luckily the small intestine of the elderly does not show many changes in old age and functions almost normally like in the young. In some individuals, however, difficulty in absorption may be noticed. Overgrowth of bacteria in the small intestine occurs in some elderly persons leading to certain symptoms like bloating or diarrhea.

The large intestine is not normally affected by aging. Constipation, however, plagues the elderly not only because of age, but also because of their lifestyle and problems with their food and liquid intake. Many medications taken by the elderly can reduce the movements of the large intestine causing constipation.

The normal human gut is populated by bacteria. These are called the *human intestinal microbiota*. These bacteria are different in the new-born infant and the young adult. As age advances, the types of bacteria in the intestines may change and this can give rise to various diseases of the GIS mainly related to the large intestine.

As one ages, various problems of the digestive tract may occur. It is estimated that about 40% of the elderly develop one or other disorders of the GIS in a year. Some of the common problems associated with the GIS are being discussed in this chapter.

DISORDERS OF THE MOUTH

The GIS begins at the mouth. Various problems may arise in the elderly in the mouth and throat due to old age. Lack of teeth and dentures may pose difficulties with chewing. Swallowing may be affected in the elderly. (See Section on *Swallowing in Book 1*). Some of the common concerns are given below.

<u>DRYNESS OF THE MOUTH</u> (*Xerostomia*)

Mild dryness of the mouth may occur in old age due to the decrease in quantity of saliva secreted. But dryness may occur as part of certain diseases and due to the side effects of medications taken for various co-existing diseases in the elderly.

Radiation to the head and neck given in certain cancers can damage the salivary glands in the mouth and cause reduction in saliva leading to dryness. Chewing of food becomes difficult in the presence of dryness.

Offending medicines if any, may be withdrawn or substituted by the physician to relieve dryness of the mouth. In others, frequent sips of any liquid or water during feeding may be needed to facilitate chewing. Salivary supplements are available and may be used. (See Chapter on *Dental Problems*).

<u>TASTE DISTURBANCES</u>

Alteration in the sense of taste or a bad taste in the mouth is called *Dysgeusia*. This may be seen in certain diseases like facial paralysis and other disorders of the nervous system. Zinc deficiency can lead to distortion of taste in the elderly as a part of malnutrition. Certain medications like those used for depression, high blood pressure, certain antibiotics and antibacterials may cause dysgeusia. The offending medicine should be removed when symptoms are present.

DISORDERS OF THE ESOPHAGUS

Aging produces mild changes in the esophagus and causes difficulty in swallowing food and liquids. Some of the common esophageal disorders of old age are described below.

ESOPHAGEAL DYSPHAGIA.

The word *'dysphagia'* denotes a difficulty in swallowing. Many conditions which occur in old age can cause difficulty in swallowing.

There may be a tumour in the esophagus or a narrowing of the esophagus (*stricture*) causing the problem. The patient feels as if food is stuck in his chest and is not going down.

There can be pressure on the esophagus inside the chest by tumors in the chest.

Inflammation of the esophagus can cause difficulty in swallowing.

In all these cases, the surgeon or the *Gastroenterologist* examines the interior of the esophagus using an *Endoscope* to determine the cause of the dysphagia and treats them appropriately. In some patients, the difficulty in swallowing is associated with pain while swallowing the food.

GASTROESOPHAGEAL REFLUX DISEASE (GERD)

This is a condition where the acid contents of the stomach flows back into the esophagus producing heartburn. (See section on *Laryngopharyngeal Reflux in ENT disorders-Book 1*) It is the most common gastrointestinal disorder in older adults. GERD is said to be prevalent in 23% of the elderly population.

What are the causes of GERD.

Some of the causes of GERD are:

- Eating foods containing excess spices like ginger, chillies, pepper, garlic etc. These increase the chances of GERD.
- Fast foods can lead to GERD in some individuals. Fried food items may cause the problem as they tend to remain in the

stomach for longer periods before being emptied into the small intestine.

- Chemical additives like Ajinomoto in food can lead to GERD.
- Going to bed soon after taking food is a common cause.
- Obese persons, especially those with abdominal obesity tend to develop the disorder.
- Certain medications cause GERD as a side effect. Medicines taken for high blood pressure, certain antibiotics, pain killers, asthma medications, steroids and sedatives can lead to GERD. These medicines weaken the ring-shaped muscle at the lower end of the esophagus (*sphincter*) which closes the esophagus tightly in normal people to prevent the reflux.
- Eating late at night and consuming alcohol or excess coffee can cause GERD.

What are the symptoms of GERD.

The commonest symptom is heart burn. The patient feels a burning sensation behind his breastbone after taking food or while lying down.

GERD very commonly causes respiratory symptoms like cough due to the acidic reflux irritating the larynx (voice box). This can trickle into the lung to cause cough and wheezing in the elderly.

Nausea and vomiting may be produced in some individuals. Belching is common. Difficulty in swallowing or painful swallowing may be experienced by some, especially if inflammation of the esophagus is present.

Some individuals have severe pain, and a heart attack may be suspected necessitating a visit to the emergency room to exclude it with an Electrocardiogram (ECG).

Weight loss and anemia may be seen in some elderly patients with GERD. Repeated bleeding from the esophagus may rarely occur leading to anemia. The presence of digested blood gives the stools of the patient a black color.

GERD can produce frequent **Esophagitis**, which is inflammation of the esophagus. This may lead to esophageal cancer in some patients.

The diagnosis of the condition is mainly by Endoscopy where the Gastroenterologist can see the whole esophagus and assess the complications of GERD. A *biopsy* of the lining of the esophagus may be taken for laboratory tests.

How is GERD treated and prevented.

The main aspects of treatment of the disease are:

- Modification of the lifestyle, weight control and avoidance of obesity are very important. Regular exercises must be undertaken by the elderly.

- If any medications are identified as the cause for GERD, they should be withdrawn by the doctor and other substitutes given.

- The patient with GERD should be advised to go to bed only after two to three hours of taking food. The head end of the bed may be raised to prevent the reflux. A couple of pillows or a board should be sufficient.

- Foods that can provoke GERD, like spicy foods, fried items and fast foods are better avoided.

- Tobacco in any form, alcohol, caffeine, citrus fruit juices like lemon and orange juice, peppermint, and fat containing foods aggravate GERD and are better excluded.

- Antacid liquids are given for treatment of GERD. They are taken three to four times a day depending on the symptoms.

- Other medications named Proton Pump Inhibitors are given by the physician to reduce the amount of acid produced in the stomach. Medications for increasing the emptying of the stomach are also effective in reducing the time the food remains in the stomach thus decreasing the chances of reflux.

- Various other treatment modalities are available like Endoscopic Surgical techniques to treat the disease. Antireflux surgery is available for treatment of GERD in the elderly.

DISORDERS OF THE STOMACH

The normal bacteria in the stomach are altered as one grows older. In addition, the lining of the stomach gradually loses its protective function and thins out. The secretion of acid in the stomach decreases as age advances. The blood flow to the stomach may be compromised in old age. The time taken for stomach to empty its contents into the intestines is delayed. All these changes lead to disorders of the stomach in old age. To add to this, the elderly have many other co-existing illnesses which necessitate the administration of various medications which can upset the stomach.

GASTRITIS AND H. PYLORI INFECTION

Gastritis implies inflammation of the inner lining of the stomach. A bacterium called *Helicobacter pylori*. (*H. pylori*) is seen in the stomach of most of the elderly people. *H. pylori* is a risk for the development of stomach cancer. These bacteria are associated with the risk of developing peptic ulcer, GERD, and other systemic illnesses like vitamin B12 deficiency, iron deficiency, Alzheimer's disease, cardiovascular disease, and thyroid abnormalities.

H. pylori can be diagnosed by various tests in the blood and *stools* of the patient. Their presence can also be detected in a *biopsy* of the stomach lining taken during endoscopy.

Clinically *H. pylori* infection can produce various symptoms. In some it may produce simple, frequent stomach upsets. In others it may produce symptoms of peptic ulcer or may even lead to stomach cancer. Nausea, vomiting, belching, and abdominal pain are seen in many patients.

H. pylori infection is treated with a regimen of a combination of antibiotics given for a period specified by the physician or *Gastroenterologist*. The symptoms may be controlled using proton pump inhibiting medications.

PEPTIC ULCER

Peptic ulcers denote ulcers that develop in the lining of the stomach and duodenum (first part of the intestine). They can occur at any age. The elderly are more prone to ulcers in the stomach.

Causes of Peptic Ulcer.

The main cause of peptic ulcer is H. pylori which has been discussed above.

The second common cause is the frequent use of pain-relieving medicines like aspirin, ibuprofen and other *NSAIDs*. Medications like steroids may cause peptic ulcer. Medicines used in heart diseases to prevent the clotting of blood (*Anticoagulants*) are known to cause peptic ulcer and increase the chances of bleeding from the ulcer.

Smoking, excess coffee, and alcohol are related to the causation of peptic ulcer.

Rarely, in some individuals the stomach produces excess gastric acid, which can lead to peptic ulcer. The disease may occur in families.

Mental stress and excess intake of highly spicy foods increases the risk of developing peptic ulcer.

What are the symptoms of peptic ulcer.

The commonest symptom is the presence of a burning pain in the pit of the stomach or upper abdomen associated with heartburn. The pain starts two or three hours after taking food. Often the pain awakens the person at night. Occasionally it may be very severe. In some persons the pain occurs at the back of the abdomen and this is seen with ulcers which occur at the back of the duodenum.

In some patients symptoms like nausea, vomiting or belching may be noted. Fullness of the stomach and a bloated feeling may be present in some individuals.

Occasionally, the ulcers may bleed. Small amounts of blood may be digested and render the stools black and sticky or tar-like. When the bleeding is profuse, the patient may suddenly vomit out the fresh blood or altered blood which looks like coffee grounds. The blood is altered by the acid in the stomach.

Repeated bleeding may cause anemia and severe tiredness in the person. Changes in the appetite of the person may be noted. The symptoms may be increased on taking fatty food.

What are the complications of Peptic Ulcer.

- Bleeding is a complication that is noted with peptic ulcer and has been discussed above.

- The ulcer can eat through the wall of the stomach and produce a hole in the stomach wall through which stomach contents and acid leak out into the *abdomen*. The patient develops excruciating abdominal pain of sudden onset. This is an emergency and calls for immediate surgical treatment.

- Over a period, the duodenal ulcers may cause narrowing of the duodenum (*stricture*) due to scarring and thereby cause a delay in emptying of the stomach. This obstruction can cause recurrent vomiting and loss of weight. The patient feels frightened to eat food for fear of vomiting and this leads to malnutrition.

- Patients with H. pylori infection and peptic ulcer can develop cancer of the stomach or duodenum later.

How is the disease diagnosed and treated.

Diagnosis of peptic ulcer has been made easy by Endoscopy where the *Gastroenterologist* passes a tube-like instrument into the stomach and visualizes the stomach and the ulcer. He can take a bit of tissue from the edge of the ulcer (*biopsy*) to see if it is cancerous and test the sample for H. pylori. Other tests for H. pylori are also available and may be done.

Occasionally, the disease is diagnosed by taking X-rays of the stomach and duodenum after drinking a liquid containing Barium Sulphate. This coats the inner wall of the stomach and this can be seen in the X-ray as an opaque shadow along with the ulcer. The test also brings out the obstruction in the stomach or duodenum caused by the ulcer.

The blood may be tested for anemia and the stools tested for the presence of digested blood if the patient has bleeding from the ulcer.

How is Peptic Ulcer treated.

The treatment of peptic ulcer is easy in modern times with the advent of many effective medications. The salient aspects of treatment are:

- The cause and risk factors for the peptic ulcer should be removed. The use of pain-relieving medications should be minimized. Alcohol and smoking should be stopped. The food intake should be more bland and excess spices avoided.
- The infection with H. pylori, if confirmed, is treated with a combination of antibiotics.
- Medications to reduce acid production are used. They are called Proton Pump inhibitors. The physician prescribes them if needed.
- Antacids are medicines that neutralize the acid in the stomach and give temporary, symptomatic relief of the pain. They are available as chewable tablets and liquids of various types. They are taken when the pain occurs. They may be taken one hour after the intake of food when the pain is expected to occur. It is not necessary to take antacids regularly and they may be used only when necessary.
- Medications are available which produce a protective coating on the inner lining of the stomach thereby preventing further damage to the lining and promote healing of the ulcer.
- Surgery of peptic ulcer was being done previously to remove a part of the stomach and attach the rest of the stomach to the small intestines. Now a days, surgery is limited to treating complications like bleeding, obstruction, and sudden rupture of the stomach due to the ulcer eroding the wall of the

stomach. The obstruction in the outlet of the stomach is bypassed by connecting the stomach directly to the duodenum or lower part of the small intestines.

What diet should be followed in Treatment and Prevention.

- The diet of the patient should be modified for the treatment of peptic ulcer disease and for its prevention. A high fiber diet with plenty of fruits and vegetables is recommended. Whole grains should be included in the diet. Fruits containing *flavonoids* and other *antioxidants* are very useful in controlling and preventing the disease. Flavonoids are found in colored fruits and vegetables like cranberries, pomegranate, strawberries, carrots, beetroot, bell pepper and broccoli.

- Garlic, onions, and green tea are useful in the prevention of peptic ulcer disease.

- Fermented *probiotic* foods like yogurt, curds and *buttermilk* are beneficial. *Probiotic* capsules may be taken on the advice of the physician. These are useful especially when an antibiotic is prescribed to treat H. pylori.

- Caffeine containing beverages, alcohol, spicy foods, pickles, *masala* containing foods, fried foods, citrus fruits, and chocolate are to be used sparingly or eschewed as these can aggravate peptic ulcer.

- Lean proteins, fish and eggs may be taken. Vegetarians should include enough lentils, beans, peas, and tofu in their diet to supplement proteins. Excess use of milk can increase stomach acid and hence is avoided or used to a minimum.

DISORDERS OF THE INTESTINES

Various disorders of the small intestines and large intestines may occur in the elderly. A few important ones are discussed below.

IRRITABLE BOWEL SYNDROME (IBS)

Irritable Bowel Syndrome (**IBS**) can present with various symptoms and is not unusual in the elderly population

What are the causes of IBS.

Even though the exact cause is not known, multiple factors have been attributed to cause IBS.

- Muscle contractions like cramps occurring in the intestines is said to lead to IBS.
- Abnormalities in the nervous system may lead to IBS by altering the signals from the brain to the intestinal tract.
- Occasionally, infections in the intestines with a heavy growth of bacteria can lead to the symptoms of IBS. In some patients, IBS may follow a bout of intestinal infection presenting as diarrhea which is often the predominant symptom.
- Mental stress can lead to exacerbation of IBS if the patient is prone to the disease. Psychological problems like anxiety and depression can present as IBS. IBS prior to examination is not uncommon in the young student.
- Various types of food allergies can provoke symptoms of IBS in an individual. These include milk, wheat, carbonated drinks, citrus fruits, juices, and legumes.
- A genetic predisposition to develop IBS exists and may be seen in children of parents with IBS.

What are the symptoms of IBS.

The symptoms may be mild or severe depending on the individual. The various symptoms are:

- Cramping stomach pains more often after food and relieved when the patient passes stools.
- Heartburn, bloating, indigestion, vomiting and an urge to pass stools frequently, even though the quantity of stools may be very little.
- Passing urine frequently.
- Some persons feel constipated even though they get the sensation to pass stools frequently. The stools may be watery with plenty of sticky, whitish *mucus*.
- Rarer symptoms include headaches, fever, loss of weight, anxiety, and severe tiredness.

How can IBS be treated.

A holistic approach to the treatment of IBS must be adopted in most patients as there is no single treatment that is effective for all patients. Some of the salient aspects in the management of IBS are given below.

- As psychological stress is a cause for IBS, especially in the elderly age group, managing stress is of paramount importance. Appropriate measures to reduce stress like meditation, yoga, exercise, and counselling are helpful in many patients. Medications to reduce stress are seldom needed and should be taken only on the advice of the physician.
- Food may be a cause of IBS in some elderly individuals. Food intolerance, not hitherto present may manifest as the person grows older. Milk, fatty and fried foods, spicy foods, citrus fruits, and root vegetables may be the cause of IBS in some. These must be identified and excluded from the diet of the elderly individual. Eating smaller meals frequently may keep the symptoms of IBS under control in some individuals.
- Regular exercise like walking, cycling, or swimming is

important in maintaining the physical and mental fitness of the person. Exercise relieves the symptoms of IBS in them.

- <u>Dietary fiber</u> intake should be ensured by increasing the intake of vegetables, fruits, nuts, and wholegrains. Whenever needed dietary fiber can be supplemented in the individual in the form of psyllium fiber, or methyl cellulose. Probiotics may be supplemented in the diet. These are to be taken on the advice of the physician. A *Gluten* free diet is prescribed to some patients to prevent the symptoms of IBS.

- <u>Smokers</u> should quit the habit. <u>Alcohol</u> intake also should be avoided or moderated.

- <u>Medications</u> are prescribed for IBS by the physician as and when needed. Mild laxatives or stool softeners may be prescribed when constipation is the predominant symptom. Medications may be needed for diarrhea.

<u>DIVERTICULOSIS</u>

Diverticular disease or *diverticulosis* is a condition where small sac-like outpouchings occur in the large intestine or colon of the person. This is a disease common in the West and other industrialized countries and less so in the developing world. These sac-like outpouchings are called *Diverticula* (Singular: *Diverticulum*). The disease is more common as one ages. It is most common in the 50-80 age group where almost 50 - 65% of persons have diverticula in their colon. Majority of these patients have no symptoms. Only about 15-20% of patients with the diverticula develop symptoms. Men and women are equally affected.

What causes Diverticular disease.

Though the cause of the disease is not known, the commonest cause attributed is the lack of fiber in the diet as seen in the Western countries and other developed countries. The people in the developing countries are used to a diet which is mainly whole grain and vegetable based containing plenty of fiber. Lack of fiber in the diet increases the time taken for the digested food to pass through the large intestine and this stagnant stool leads to the development of diverticula.

Other causes attributed to the causation of the disease are *spasm* occurring in the muscles of the large intestine, obesity, lack of regular exercise and some medications which may cause the disease.

What are the symptoms of the disease.

- Majority of the individuals with diverticula in their colon have no symptoms.
- The small percentage of individuals with symptoms may complain of pain in the left side of the abdomen. The pain may be of a cramping nature and severe in some. The affected area of the abdomen maybe painful to touch.
- In some patients, these diverticula become infected with bacteria. This condition is called *Diverticulitis.*
- Diverticulitis is often associated with fever, nausea, diarrhea and severe tiredness. Others may develop loss of appetite and loss of weight.
- Occasionally, these infected diverticula can burst causing the infection to spread into the cavity of the abdomen leading to severe infection of the peritoneum called *Peritonitis.* This can be dangerous and occasionally fatal in the elderly age group.
- Occasionally bleeding can occur from the diverticula causing bright red blood to be seen along with stools. This may be painless in some.
- Severe diverticulitis may subsequently cause scarring in the large intestine leading to obstruction in the bowel. This is called *Stricture* of the colon and leads to resistant constipation in the patient.

How is Diverticular disease diagnosed.
There are many methods of diagnosing the disease.

- *Barium enema* is a simple X-ray test which is done. A liquid containing Barium sulphate solution is passed into the colon through a tube as an *enema*. The liquid lines the inner wall of the colon and delineates the diverticula. This can be seen on X-rays of the abdomen.

- Another test done is *Colonoscopy*, where an *Endoscope* is introduced into the colon from below and the interior of the colon is viewed by the Gastroenterologist. The diverticula can be visualized in this test.

- A *Computerized Tomography (CT) Scan* of the abdomen shows the large intestine and the diverticula clearly and helps to diagnose the condition.

- *Ultrasound Scan* is useful in the diagnosing diverticulosis.

- *Magnetic Resonance Imaging (MRI)* is another diagnostic test that gives very good images of the colon for the Gastroenterologist to make a comprehensive diagnosis.

How is Diverticular Disease treated.

Treatment of Diverticular disease comprises prevention of infection in the diverticula (diverticulitis), treatment of acute pain and infection when they occur and tackling the complications of the disease. The main aspects of treatment are as follows:

- Preventing infection occurring in those with no symptoms is important. The diet should contain enough fibers in the form of vegetables and fruits. For some patients fiber supplements will be needed. Commercial preparation of fiber supplements like psyllium and methyl cellulose are available. The main aim is to prevent constipation in the elderly individual.

- Antibiotics are prescribed by the *Gastroenterologist* for the control of the infection in diverticulitis.

- *Probiotics* are of help to increase the favourable bacteria in the intestines. This is helpful in some individuals with symptoms of diarrhea and bloating.

- <u>Pain relief</u> can be achieved with medications that relieve the spasm of the intestines.
- <u>Surgery</u> is needed in some patients where a portion of the large intestine is removed.
- <u>Complications</u> of the disease may need hospitalization and surgery.

CONSTIPATION

Constipation is the condition where there is difficulty in emptying the bowels associated with hardened stools. Every individual at some point in their life would have had this symptom. But when this is recurrent and chronic, it becomes an annoying problem. Elderly persons are more likely to develop constipation and it has been found that of the older people living in nursing homes about 50% have chronic constipation.

Many factors can cause constipation. Some of the causes are elaborated below.

- A <u>diet low in fiber</u> is the commonest cause. It is seen in elderly persons confined to bed. The elderly who live alone may have a lack of interest in eating and drinking fluids and this can lead to constipation.
- A <u>decrease in water intake</u> by the elderly person is an important cause. (See Section on *Dehydration in Book 1*).
- Elderly individuals may be on <u>multiple medications</u> for various illnesses and the side effects of these medications may be a cause of constipation. Medications containing codeine, like certain cough remedies, opiates, calcium preparations, allergy medications, sedatives, and medications given for abdominal pain and cramps may cause constipation.
- <u>Electrolyte imbalances</u>, <u>endocrine diseases</u> like hypothyroidism, and various diseases of the nervous system

may lead to constipation.

- <u>Mechanical obstruction</u> to movement of stools in the intestines like tumors or strictures causing obstruction, may cause constipation.
- Patients with anxiety, depression and other <u>psychiatric problems</u> often are constipated.
- <u>Lack of exercise</u> is an important cause of constipation in the elderly. Sedentary individuals have a higher incidence of constipation.
- Other causes are a <u>lax abdominal wall</u> due to obesity or multiple pregnancies in women. Weakness of the pelvic muscles may occur in women following multiple pregnancies.

Symptoms of Constipation.

The symptoms of constipation vary depending on its severity.

A normal person usually empties his bowels once daily. Some have bowel movements only 4 to 5 times a week. This is also normal. When a person has not passed stools for 3 days consecutively, constipation should be suspected.

Other symptoms like loss of appetite, mild pain at the lower back, general tiredness, a feeling of bloating in the abdomen, abdominal discomfort, and a sensation of not having emptied the bowels completely, are common symptoms. The stools are hard and lumpy, and the person feels the need to strain excessively to pass stools.

Some elderly patients become irritable and constipation may not be suspected as a cause of their behaviour.

Occasionally, the stools get dried up into a hard mass in the rectum and causes severe constipation with pain. This is called *'fecal impaction'* and may cause severe abdominal discomfort.

If blood which is bright red or tarry in color is noticed in stools, more serious causes like tumors should be suspected and prompt medical advice sought.

Prevention and Management of Constipation.

Lifestyle and Diet. Changes in lifestyle are important in the prevention and management of constipation in the elderly. The patient is encouraged to be active as much as possible. Exercises like yoga and other abdominal exercises performed in the mornings aids easy evacuation.

- The patient should be encouraged to have a regular schedule for passing stools. Post breakfast toileting is ideal. This can be developed into a habit by daily practice. The person is advised to walk about for ten minutes to get the feeling to pass stools. This type of bowel training is important. The movement of the large intestine is maximum during the morning hours and the bowel training to pass stools during this time is important. A hot cup of tea or coffee or a cup or two of warm water in the morning aids bowel movements in some individuals.

- Using a foot stool to raise the feet or using a semi-squatting posture while passing stools aids better clearance. The Indian habit of squatting for stools is one of the best methods to avoid constipation and pass stools effortlessly.

- The elderly individual should not ignore and withhold the urge to pass stools.

- The diet should include adequate fiber. An adult needs 20-35 grams of fiber and 1.5 – 2 liters of liquid per day. This should be given in the form of fruits and vegetables to prevent constipation. Prunes are very useful in treating and preventing constipation. Other fiber containing foods are oats, peas, beans, whole wheat bran, whole wheat bread, and nuts. Two to four tablespoonful raw bran may be taken with each meal along with a glass of water.

Medications. Medications are used when the lifestyle and diet management fail to correct the constipation.

- Laxatives are the most used preparations to treat constipation. Various types of laxatives are available. They may be taken as advised by the physician. Over the counter preparations of laxatives are available and should be taken after carefully reading the instructions given on the label.

- Bulk forming agents like psyllium and methyl cellulose are given as fiber supplements. They increase the bulk of the stools by absorbing water and thereby keeping the stools soft and easily passable.

- *Probiotics* are helpful in preventing and treating constipation in the elderly. Natural probiotics like yogurt, curds and *buttermilk* may be included in the diet daily.

- When the stools have hardened in the rectum, an enema may be given to soften the stools and help easy emptying. *Suppositories* are useful instead of enemas and can be used by the patients themselves.

- Rarely when they have formed into a hard solid mass which cannot pass through the anus normally, manual removal of impacted stools may be needed by a trained person.

CANCER OF THE GASTORINTESTINAL SYSTEM

Cancers can affect any part of the Gastrointestinal system. The two common cancers discussed here are cancer of the stomach and colon (large intestine).

CANCER OF THE STOMACH

Cancer of the stomach or *Gastric Cancer* is the fifth common cancer in the world and is the third commonest cause of cancer death in the world. It is more common above the age of 65.

The symptoms of stomach cancer are as follows.

- In the early stages, stomach cancer may have no symptoms. Occasionally the patient feels a vague discomfort in the upper part of the abdomen. The person may feel indigestion. As the cancer increases in size, the person may feel pain in the stomach on taking food. Occasionally difficulty in swallowing is felt especially when the cancer is in the upper portion of the stomach.
- Loss of appetite is often an important symptom. The person may find it difficult to eat and stops eating food after a few mouthfuls. Occasionally, they may not eat for days together and end up losing weight. The person feels 'full' even after eating very little.
- The stools may be black or 'tarry' due to the presence of digested blood from the cancer. This is a warning sign and must be investigated immediately.
- Some patients feel nausea and may vomit occasionally after taking food. The color may be coffee-ground if there is blood in the vomited content.
- Excess tiredness may be felt due to undernourishment and anemia. The repeated bleeding and loss of blood may result in

anemia.

- Some patients may have a low-grade fever associated with the cancer.
- Patients who have had peptic ulcer infected with H. pylori may develop stomach cancer. The symptoms of peptic ulcer are present in them.

The **Causes and Risk** of cancer are also known.

- Men are more prone to stomach cancer than women.
- Increasing age increases the risk of developing the cancer.
- Smokers are twice more likely to develop stomach cancer.
- H. Pylori infection has been shown to develop into cancer later in life.
- A diet high in meat and pickles has been shown to increase the risk.
- A family history of cancer is important as it may be seen in family members. This could be due to genetic transmission of the cancer.
- Previous surgery on the stomach and peptic ulcers may increase the risk of developing stomach cancer.

The cancer may spread to nearby structures in the abdomen like the liver, pancreas, intestines, and *peritoneum*. It may spread to the *lymph nodes* in the abdomen and spread through blood to remote organs like the lungs and the brain. This type of spread to other organs through blood is called *Metastasis* of the cancer.

Diagnosis. The disease is diagnosed by performing an Endoscopy where the endoscope is introduced into the stomach through the mouth and the interior of the stomach is visualized by the Gastroenterologist. A biopsy of the tumor is taken for microscopic analysis. This confirms the type of cell causing the cancer and aids in planning the treatment.

Ultrasound Scan of the abdomen helps in diagnosing the cancer and the presence of lymph node enlargement. The spread of the cancer to nearby organs can be identified by ultrasound scan.

A Barium X-ray can be used to diagnose the condition. The patient drinks a liquid containing barium and X-rays of the abdomen are taken. The barium in the stomach delineates the cancer clearly.

Other tests like CT scan or *Positron Emission Tomography (PET scan)* are used to know the location and extent of the cancer and whether it has spread to nearby organs and distant areas of the body.

How is stomach cancer treated.

The three main treatment methods for stomach cancer are Surgery, Chemotherapy and Radiation Treatment.

<u>Surgery</u> is the main mode of treatment. Various types of surgery are done to remove the cancer in the stomach. Occasionally, surgery of the stomach is combined with removal of the lymph nodes around it if they have been invaded by the cancer cells.

<u>Radiation therapy</u> is used after surgery to destroy any residual cancer cells present. Sometimes radiation is given along with chemotherapy.

<u>Chemotherapy</u> is given either before or after the surgery. When it is given before the surgery, it shrinks the tumor and makes the surgery easier to perform. It may be given after surgery to kill any residual cancer cells that may be present. Often, surgery, radiation and chemotherapy are combined in a patient. Chemotherapy is given in cycles giving a gap between two cycles.

<u>Targeted Therapy</u> is another method of treatment of cancer where specific medications are used to target only the cancer cells. <u>Immunotherapy</u> uses medications to stimulate the person's own immune system to find and destroy the cancer cells.

The type of treatment to be given is decided by a team which consists of the Gastroenterologist, the Surgeon, and the *Oncologist.*

In addition to the specific treatment of the cancer, other measures to improve the nutrition of the patient, treat the anemia and control the symptoms and side effects of treatment are also given to the patient.

CANCER OF THE COLON

Colon cancer occurs in the large intestine. It is also called Colorectal Cancer (**CRC**) as it often affects the large intestine and the rectum. The cancer is one of the commonest types worldwide and affects the elderly much more than the young. Its incidence is almost 50% in those above the age of 80. Every year about 150,000 Americans are detected to have CRC.

What are the risks for developing CRC.

Many factors have been identified in the development of CRC. Some of these are:

- <u>Age</u> of the person is important. CRC is a disease of the elderly. 70% of CRC is seen in individuals above the age of 65.

- <u>Men</u> have a higher rate of CRC than women.
- <u>African Americans</u> have a higher rate of developing CRC.
- A <u>family history</u> of CRC is important. Close relatives of patients with CRC have a higher risk of getting the disease.
- Persons with certain <u>inflammatory diseases</u> of the bowel run the risk of developing CRC.
- Some patients who are at risk of CRC may have small growths called *Polyps* arising from the inner lining of the large intestines. They may be multiple. These are *benign* growths with a small stalk and are 5-10 millimetre in size. Large polyps may turn cancerous.
- <u>Obesity and lack of exercise</u> are important risk factors. A sedentary life increases the risk of CRC.
- <u>Smokers</u> are said to be at a higher risk of developing the cancer. <u>Alcohol</u> is a risk factor.
- <u>Excess use of red meat and processed meat</u> is mentioned as

a risk factor. Too much <u>fat in diet</u> with low fiber content increases the risk for developing the disease.

- <u>Diabetics</u> have a higher risk of developing CRC.
- <u>Previous Radiation treatment</u> to the lower abdomen for any cause can lead to CRC development later in life.

What are the symptoms of CRC.

Some of the common symptoms that are associated with CRC are:

- A change in a person's bowel habits like diarrhea or constipation which occurs despite the individual taking a normal diet. The stools may be thin and ribbon like.
- The presence of blood in stools.
- Excess weakness and loss of weight. This may be due to the anemia which the patient develops following the loss of blood.
- The person feels discomfort in the lower part of the abdomen along with cramps.
- There is a feeling that he has not emptied the bowel completely even after passing stools.

How can CRC be prevented.

Many preventive measures have been advocated.

- Lifestyle modification is the most important preventive measure that must be adopted early in life. A wholesome diet consisting of fruits, vegetables, nuts along with vitamins and minerals is necessary for prevention. Use of red and processed meat should be limited.
- Regular exercise should be made part of one's lifestyle.
- Alcohol consumption should be moderated. The permitted alcohol intake is two drinks a day for men and one for women.
- Weight control is of prime importance in preventing CRC. Persons with a family history of the disease should be careful

to control their weight.

- Quitting smoking is important.
- The use of aspirin in the prevention of CRC has been described in some studies. But it should be taken only after consultation with one's physician.

Diagnosis of CRC.

Screening for CRC is done after the age of 45. Persons at a higher risk of developing the disease are screened more frequently. If polyps are found at screening, they are removed. Stools are tested during screening.

Colonoscopy is the endoscopy for looking into the colon. The Gastroenterologist passes the endoscope from below through the anus and examines the inside of the colon to see if there are any growths or bleeding areas in the colon. Polyps, if present can be removed during endoscopy. Biopsy is taken from the colon if the doctor suspects cancer.

Other tests like CT scans or PET scans may be ordered by the doctor if *metastasis* to other areas is suspected. Ultrasound scan of the abdomen is done as a part of the investigation.

How is CRC treated.

Surgery is the treatment of choice for CRC. The type of surgery will depend on the size of the cancer and whether it has spread. A part of the colon may be removed during surgery. The lymph nodes surrounding the colon may be removed if they are affected.

Chemotherapy, Radiation Therapy, Targeted Therapy, and Immunotherapy may be planned for the person depending on the type of CRC and its spread to other organs.

When the disease is far advanced, palliative treatment is advised to improve the quality of life of the patient and make his remaining days comfortable and free of pain and symptoms.

Resources.

1. Davidson's Principles and Practice of Medicine. 23rd Edition. Elsevier

2018. Chapter 21. *Gastroenterology* pages 763 – 844.

2. Gastrointestinal Tract Disorders in Old Age. Dumic I et al. *Canadian J. of Gastroenterology & Hepatology.* 2019, Vol 2019. Pages 1-19.

https://www.ncbi.nlm.nih.gov/pmc/articles/PMC6354172/

1. Gastroesophageal Reflux Disease. Important considerations for older patients. Chait MM. *World J. of Gastrointestinal Endoscopy.* 2010. 2: 388-396.

https://www.ncbi.nlm.nih.gov/pmc/articles/PMC3010469/

1. Disorders of the Digestive System in the Elderly. Shamburek RD, Farrar JT. *New Engl. J. Med.* 1990. 322: pages 438-443

https://www.nejm.org/doi/full/10.1056/NEJM199002153220705

1. Irritable Bowel Syndrome (IBS) in Elderly Adults. Rodríguez J. *Griswold Home Care.* 2022.

https://www.griswoldhomecare.com/blog/2022/august/irritable-bowel-syndrome-ibs-in-elderly-adults/

1. Peptic Ulcer. *Mayo Clinic* 2022.

https://www.mayoclinic.org/diseases-conditions/peptic-ulcer/symptoms-causes/syc-20354223

1. Diverticular Disease in the Elderly. Comparato G et al. *Digestive Diseases* 2007. 25 : pages 151-159

https://www.karger.com/Article/Pdf/99480

1. Management of Constipation in Older Adults. Mounsey A et al. *Amer. Fam. Physician.* 2015. 92: pages. 500-504

https://www.aafp.org/pubs/afp/issues/2015/0915/p500.html

1. Colorectal Cancer treatment in Older Patients. Sanoff HK, Goldberg RM. *Gastrointest Cancer Res*. 2007 1 : pages 248-253

https://www.ncbi.nlm.nih.gov/pmc/articles/PMC2631216/

1. Colon Cancer. *Mayo Clinic. 2022*

https://www.mayoclinic.org/diseases-conditions/colon-cancer/symptoms-causes/syc-20353669

2. THE SKIN

Of all the organs in the body, the skin is the largest as it covers the whole body and occupies a large surface area. The skin occupies an area of about 20 square feet in an average sized man. The main functions of the skin are **Protection, Regulation and Sensation.**

- The skin protects the whole body from external injury and substances.
- It protects the body from Ultraviolet radiation from the sun's rays.
- It helps in the regulation of body temperature.
- The skin helps to retain moisture inside the body.
- It contains the sense organs of touch, pain and temperature which detect these sensations.
- The skin produces Vitamin D when exposed to natural sunlight.
- It protects the body against infections as bacteria and viruses cannot freely penetrate the unbroken skin.

<u>**Parts of the Skin.**</u>

The skin has three main parts known as the **Epidermis, Dermis** and **Hypodermis** or Subcutaneous Tissue. The thickness and texture of the skin is different in different parts of the body. The skin of the palms and soles is very thick compared to the skin of the eyelids.

EPIDERMIS. This is the outermost layer of skin and is formed of cells that contain a protein called Keratin. The Epidermis provides the outer protective layer of the skin.

There is another type of cell in the epidermis which contains a pigment called *Melanin*, which provides the color to the skin.

A third type of cells are present in the epidermis which ward off infections and fight bacteria.

The epidermis continuously produces new cells as the old worn out cells are shed daily. Hence, the cells on the surface of the skin are dead cells. The surface of the epidermis contains numerous *pores* or tiny openings of the sweat glands and hair follicles. (Figure 2)

DERMIS. The dermis is the middle layer which lies below the epidermis. It occupies a major part of the skin's structure. The Dermis is made up of many structures.

Collagen and Elastin which are proteins give the skin their flexibility and strength.

The dermis contains blood vessels which supply blood to the skin.

Nerves and small nerve endings which help in detecting touch, pain, and temperature changes are present in the dermis.

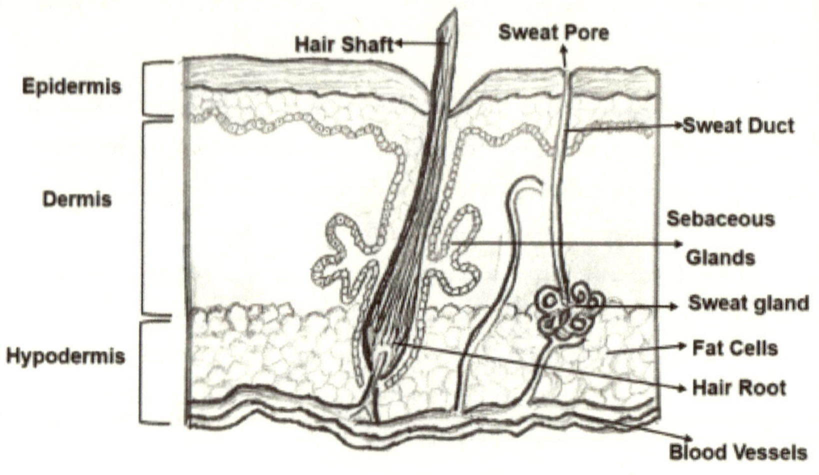

Figure 2

Certain glands named Sebaceous glands are present in the dermis. They secrete an oily substance called Sebum which keeps the surface of the skin soft, smooth, and lubricated. These are more numerous and larger over the forehead, around the nose, mouth, and cheeks. Excess sebum secretion causes the oily skin in some individuals.

Sweat glands present in the dermis produce sweat which reaches the surface of the skin (epidermis) through small ducts.

The dermis contains *Hair Follicles* which give rise to the hairs which protrude on the surface of the skin.

HYPODERMIS (SUBCUTANEOUS LAYER). The word *cutaneous* indicates 'of the skin'. 'Hypo' means 'beneath'. Hence Hypodermis denotes the layer beneath the dermis.

This layer is composed mainly of fatty tissue. Its thickness varies from person to person and it gives the contour to the body. The subcutaneous tissue layer protects the underlying muscles and bones. It cushions the body and provides energy to the body from the fat contained in the fat cells. The fat acts as an insulation against temperature variations. It contains the blood vessels and nerves which pass into the dermis.

NAILS. The nail is a part of the skin. It is formed of very thick compact cells which contain the protein Keratin. The main action of the nails in humans is to protect the fingertips. They provide support to the tips of the fingers to help functions like touching and grasping.

The visible part of the nail at the fingertip is called the Nail plate. It is firmly fixed on the underlying fingertip called the Nail bed. The base of the nail contains the root of the nail which is underneath the skin. It produces the cells containing keratin which grow forward and become compacted to produce the nails.

Various diseases can produce changes in the nails and these can be detected by the physician on examining the nails of the patient.

The skin is the largest organ in the human body. It functions as a barrier between the inside of the body and the external world. It helps us in regulating temperature, maintaining the *homeostasis*, proper hydration of the body and protects the body against infection. As a person gets older, the skin undergoes many changes most of which are not preventable. But factors like lifestyle, habits, heredity, and diet do influence the changes that occur in the skin as we grow older.

As one ages, the functions of the skin deteriorate. The skin becomes delicate and fragile and prone to damage by external factors like physical and chemical agents. Approximately, 25-50% of elderly persons around the world have fragile skin.

What happens to the skin as we age.

Many changes happen in the skin as we grow old. These changes make the skin prone for infections and damage by external factors. The skin in the elderly can be damaged due to external causes like exposure to sunlight, environmental causes, pollution, dust, wind etc. Some of the changes are:

- The skin becomes thinner as we age and more prone to tearing and injury. The fat below the dermis of the skin decreases with age and this can lead to easy bruising as the cushioning effect of fat is no longer present as in the skin of the young.

- As the immunity of the body decreases with age, the skin becomes unable to act as an effective barrier against infection and infections become common.
- Healing of the skin after any damage or surgery takes more time in the elderly.
- The surface of the skin becomes furrowed and wrinkled as age advances and the softness of the skin decreases. This is due to loss of elasticity of the skin.
- The exposure of the human body to ultraviolet light (sunlight) during life gradually tells upon the skin and causes most of the damage to the skin.
- The skin of an elderly individual becomes more sensitive to irritant substances compared to the young skin and is easily damaged. Detergents and other cleaning products tend to harm the skin of the elderly very easily.
- The fragility of the skin can lead to pressure sores, itching, infections of the skin and dryness of the skin.
- The presence of *co-morbidities* like diabetes and other *autoimmune diseases* can make the skin more vulnerable to fungal infections.
- Many drugs which are administered in old age for various diseases can cause changes in the skin.
- The skin around the genitals may be damaged and infected in those in whom urinary incontinence is present.
- In addition, the loss of elasticity of the skin causes a tendency of the skin to sag especially in the cheeks, below the eyes and neck. *Freckles* and dark spots tend to appear in the skin with aging.

Some of the common skin conditions that occur in old age are being discussed below.

DRY SKIN (Xerosis)

Dry skin (*Xerosis*) is one of the commonest problems of old age. It is due to the loss of water from the skin and the decrease in oil-producing glands and sweat glands in the skin which leads to reduction of the moisture held by the skin.

What are the causes of a Dry Skin.

- The skin tends to become dry by external factors like heat from room heaters, air conditioning, wind, use of irritant soaps and hot baths. Excess cleansing of the skin using soap can lead to dryness.
- Using products that dry the skin like alcohol (hand sanitizers) and frequent use of soap.
- Hypothyroidism causes dry skin.
- Certain medications cause dryness of the skin.
- Skin diseases like *Psoriasis* and *Eczema*.
- Systemic diseases like Diabetes and Chronic Kidney Disease.
- Inadequate intake of fluids leading to dehydration causes dry skin.

The symptoms of dry skin are mainly itching. The skin becomes tight and flaky. The changes are seen more on the legs (shins) and arms. The skin may be cracked and have scratch marks due to itching. Scratching may lead to infections in the skin by introducing germs into the wound.

Treatment and Prevention of Dry Skin.

- Causes for dry skin should be found and averted. Products containing Sodium Lauryl Sulphate, Alcohol, Triclosan, Lye or fragrance, should be avoided.
- Coconut oil and Sunflower oil may be massaged into the skin

after bathing to retain moisture. This is especially useful in the legs.

- Using Oatmeal powder, Bengal Gram powder and Peas powder as a scrub while bathing instead of soap is useful. This is commonly used in Asian countries, especially in South India. The South Indians take a bath after smearing the whole body with oil (usually, coconut oil or medicated *Ayurvedic* oils) and massage the skin. The individual bathes after half an hour allowing the skin to absorb most of the oil. The rest of the oil is removed by scrubbing gently with a paste made from one of the powders mentioned above and water. Soap is not used. This is the traditional **"Oil Bath"** of the South Indians. It is a very invigorating experience, especially in winter.

- Application of honey as a *moisturizer* is found to be effective.

- Moisturizer should be applied to the skin soon after bathing. A good moisturizer containing glycerin or urea is ideal. It may be applied at night before retiring to bed if the dryness is severe. Otherwise, once a day application after bath suffices.

- Alcohol based cleansers which may irritate the skin and remove the oils in the skin are better avoided. "Moisturizing Cleansers or Soaps" are useful.

- Gentle *exfoliation* of the skin may be done after bath using a towel to remove the flakes, followed by application of a moisturizer.

- It is preferable to avoid a <u>hot shower</u>. Cool and lukewarm water for bathing is ideal and helps to retain moisture in the skin. Hot showers tend to remove the normal moisture barrier of the skin. Avoid harsh, irritating, and medicated soaps. Bathing should be of only 5 – 7 minutes duration. Bathing for a longer duration tends to remove the oils from the skin.

- A healthy diet is an essential part of keeping the skin hydrated and healthy. Ensure a balanced diet with adequate vitamins and nutrients. (See section on *Nutritional Requirements* in Book 1 of the series). Always ensure that one is hydrated by drinking adequate quantity of water and other liquids.

- During winter, special care should be taken to keep the skin moist. A humidifier should be used in the room to prevent evaporation of moisture from the skin. Wearing a scarf, cap and gloves prevents the skin from drying. Vaseline should be applied to the lips to prevent dry and chapped lips.
- Excess exposure to sun's heat leads to dryness of skin.
- In spite of the home care, if the skin is still dry and itchy, one must consult a Physician or a *Dermatologist* for appropriate treatment.

The elderly should consult a physician or a Dermatologist if there is cracking of the skin with bleeding, infection, oozing from the skin or peeling of the skin.

PRESSURE SORES

Pressure sores, pressure ulcers, or bed sores, also called *Decubitus Ulcers* are common in the elderly. Those who are at a higher risk of developing them are malnourished patients, paralyzed patients, bedridden and wheel chair bound patients, cancer patients, diabetics, patients with incontinence, and critical care patients. Obese patients are more vulnerable for pressure sores.

These ulcers tend to occur over the part of the skin where there is a prominent underlying bone as in the elbows, ankles, buttocks, heels, back of the head, shoulder blades, and low back. Patients over the age of 70 are more vulnerable for bedsores. Prolonged pressure over the area leads to reduced blood flow to the skin causing damage due to lack of blood flow which nourishes the skin.

What are the symptoms of Pressure Sores

Initially, the skin may show a discoloration as red patches (in fair skinned individuals) or blue or purple patches (in the dark skinned). The skin may become warm to touch and thickened. The person may feel itching or a burning sensation at the site. This leads to *blister* formation or breaking down to create an *ulcer*. The ulcer may increase in size and depth and occasionally may involve the underlying muscle and bone. If the ulcer gets infected, pus formation is seen and the patient may develop fever. The pain may often be severe in certain individuals.

How are Pressure ulcers treated.

- The ulcers have to be dressed frequently and kept covered. Dressings are applied to accelerate the healing process.
- Specially designed dynamic mattresses are used to relieve the pressure on the affected area. These mattresses have air cells that alternatively inflate and deflate thereby reducing the pressure on the area. This helps faster healing of the ulcer.

Once formed, a bedsore takes a long time to heal, especially in patients with diabetes or other *immunocompromised* states.

- The patient's position should be frequently changed to avoid pressure over bony points in the body.
- A healthy and nutritious diet is important and adequate protein intake should be ensured.
- The surgeon cleans the wound, removes any damaged tissues and dresses up the wound.
- Antibiotics are given if the wound is infected. This is done after taking a *swab* from the wound for *culturing* the bacteria that cause the infection.
- When the wound is very extensive, the surgeon may opt for grafting healthy normal skin over the damaged area after the infection is fully under control.

What precautions are needed to prevent bed sores.

Preventing bed sores is more important, as once they set in, cure can take weeks or months in some individuals. The main preventive measures are as follows:

- Bedridden patients should be turned and repositioned every 2 or 3 hours. Those who can move by themselves should be encouraged to do so as frequently as possible. Patients on a wheelchair should change position every 15 minutes.
- Soft pillows or foam cushions may be used to keep areas pressure free. The dynamic mattresses may be used to relieve the pressure on these areas. Specially designed dynamic mattresses may be used for those at risk of developing bed sores.
- Soft paddings may be provided in beds and wheelchairs to prevent pressure on bony points.
- Care should be taken to keep the skin clean and dry.
- Good nutrition is an essential part of prevention and adequate

vitamins, minerals and proteins should be made available in the diet. Dietary supplements may be given when needed.

- Gentle massage with an oil like coconut oil is effective in preventing bedsores. One should be careful to avoid applying excess pressure during massage. Once ulceration has occurred, massage should be avoided.

- In patients at risk of pressure sores, the skin should be inspected daily for any redness or rashes and early action instituted if any change in skin color is detected.

- Other general measures to prevent pressure ulcers are prevention of smoking and controlling systemic illnesses like diabetes and high blood pressure. Obese subjects must strive to reduce weight.

SKIN INFECTIONS

Various types of infections of the skin due to bacteria, fungus and viruses may occur in the elderly population. Some of the common skin infections are discussed in this section.

BACTERIAL INFECTIONS

Various types of bacteria can cause skin infection. Of these, Staphylococci are a type of bacteria that are common in elderly subjects. These bacteria also called 'Staph' for short are commonly present in the skin and in the nose of individuals. Normally, they cause no problems. But when the skin is breached or if they enter deep into the skin or body, they can lead to serious infections.

The elderly who are at a high risk of developing skin infections are:

- Diabetics and patients with Chronic Kidney Disease.
- Immunocompromised patients like those who are on chemotherapy for cancer and patients with diseases like AIDS.
- Elderly who have dry skin and itching where the break in the skin due to scratching can lead to infection with bacteria.
- Patients who have undergone any organ transplantation.
- Burns can get infected with bacteria and cause serious illness.
- Wounds caused by injuries or surgery get infected if care is not taken to keep them clean.

The skin infections caused by Staph can be of various types. They are described in brief.

- **Boils** are the commonest of Staph infections. They are infections occurring in the sweat glands or oil producing glands of the skin. They start as reddish swelling in the skin, later on showing a yellow center due to the collection of pus.

This may break down to release the pus. Boils can be painful. They tend to occur in areas with more sweat glands like the groin, buttocks, or the arm pit.

- **Impetigo** is another condition. These are larger swellings and contain a honey-colored fluid. They may break open and form a crust. The fluid in the swelling teems with bacteria and can infect others.

- **Cellulitis** involves a larger area and the deeper layers of the skin. It is more serious. The skin is sore, swollen, painful and red. It is often seen in the legs but may occur in the face, arms, or other parts of the body. The skin may show multiple areas oozing a straw-colored liquid. Cellulitis may be associated with fever and tiredness. Diabetics are more prone for cellulitis.

Staphylococcal infections are contagious and can be transferred from one person to another through personal contact or objects like clothes, bed linen, bath towels, and other objects.

Treatment of the skin infection should be done on the advice from a doctor. Simple mild infections can be treated by applying an antibiotic skin ointment or cream to the infected area. The pain may be relieved by soothing the skin with cold compresses. When the infection is severe as in multiple boils or cellulitis, oral or injectable antibiotics may be needed. Presence of fever, chills and other symptoms may necessitate hospitalization and treatment with antibiotic injections. The physician will decide on the appropriate treatment depending on the severity of the condition.

Prevention of Skin Infections.

The salient points in the prevention of any skin infection are discussed below.

1. <u>Hand Washing</u>. This is the most important aspect in preventing any infection. The hands should be washed with

soap and water for at least 20 seconds. The fingers, the space between the fingers and the nails should be scrubbed thoroughly while washing. Hand washing should be done before taking food, after using the toilet, whenever the hands are soiled, and after touching animals or animal waste. An alcohol based sanitizer may be applied to the hands if hand washing is not possible. Hand washing should be undertaken by the caregiver of an elderly person every time he or she touches the person to help them. The elderly should take care to keep the nails of the fingers clipped short.

2. <u>Personal items</u>. Personal items like razors, towels, handkerchiefs, bed sheets and pillows should not be shared with others because bacteria may be transmitted from person to person through them.

3. <u>Wounds</u>. Any wound or break in the skin should be washed thoroughly with soap and water and kept dry or covered with a band-aid.

4. <u>Gloves</u>. Wearing of gloves during rough working or gardening should be advised to prevent injuries and pricks to the skin.

5. <u>Sanitary napkins & Tampon</u>. These should be changed frequently when they are soiled to prevent damage to the skin and subsequent infection. In bed ridden patients, preventing bed sores is important (see section on *Pressure Sores*).

6. <u>Washing clothes</u>. Bed linen and clothes used by the elderly should be washed frequently. Under garments should be changed and washed daily. In hot weather, cotton clothes should be provided to the elders as sweating can macerate the skin and lead to infection by bacteria or fungus. In tropical countries, sunshine is the best disinfecting agent and clothes may be dried in the sun. Ironing the clothes helps prevent transmission of infection.

FUNGAL INFECTIONS

Fungus is a spore producing organism we see in molds and mushrooms. It is present in plants, soil and on the surface of the skin in some individuals. There are more than a million of types of fungi of which only a few have been known to infect man. Skin infections with fungus occurs when the skin is wet with sweat as in the armpits, folds of skin, between the toes, groin and below the breasts in females. Many types of fungal infections of the skin exist. A few of the common infections seen in elderly individuals are discussed below.

What are the Risk Factors for Fungal Infections of skin.

Several factors can cause an elderly person's skin to be infected with Fungi. Some of these are as follows:

- Excess sweating is a common risk factor for fungal skin infection. Hot climates like the tropics with excess humidity in the air makes people more prone for fungal infections of the skin.

- Wearing tight clothing especially the clothes made of synthetic fabrics is another reason. This tends to cause excess sweating which is retained on the surface of the skin.

- Skin which is not kept clean and dry is a risk factor like in those working in the fields without footwear as seen in the Asian countries. People like washermen, farmers and gardeners who work with water continuously tend to get fungal infection of the feet or nails.

- Using adult diapers in bed ridden patients and in those with diseases like Alzheimer's disease tends to macerate the skin around the groin and genitals leading to fungal infections.

- Fungal infections of the skin can be transferred from animals to man due to close contact with them.

- A weak immune system as occurs during the treatment of cancer, AIDS, or use of *immunosuppressant drugs*.

- Obesity is a risk factor as the sweat is retained in the folds of the skin in these persons. Areas below the breasts in females, groins, and armpits in the obese are prone to fungal infections of the skin.

<u>Ringworm</u>

Contrary to the name, this is a fungal infection of the skin and occurs in the skin of the body, arm, neck, and legs. The medical term is *Tinea Corporis.* The skin shows itchy, red rashes which are ring-shaped. Hence the name. These rashes are slightly raised at the margins and spread outwards like a ring increasing in size as the disease spreads.

Multiple areas in the skin of the body and limbs may be affected. It is contagious. The name of the infection varies depending on the part of the body that is infected,. For e.g., *Tinea cruris* (groin), *Tinea pedis* (feet), *Tinea capitis* (scalp), *Tinea manuum* (hand) and *Tinea unguium* (nails).

The physician takes scrapings from the lesion and examines them under the microscope to see the filaments of the fungus. The fungus can be cultured in the laboratory.

How is fungal skin infection treated.

Various creams, ointments and solutions are available for treatment of the infection. They should be applied twice daily for two to three weeks till complete cure is ensured. When the skin is extensively involved as in patients who are immunocompromised or diabetic, oral preparations of anti-fungal medications are prescribed by the physician or Dermatologist. These should be given for two to four weeks.

How to prevent fungal infections of the skin.

Some important aspects of prevention of fungal infections of the skin are given below.

- Good personal hygiene is the best way to prevent infections of the skin in the elderly.
- Clothing worn should not be too tight. Cotton clothing is ideal instead of the synthetic fabrics.
- Clothes, especially innerwear should never be shared.

Innerwear should always be of cotton. Towels, handkerchiefs, and other personal items should not be shared with others.

- Shoes should not be too tight. Socks should be changed frequently. Cotton socks are desirable. After prolonged wearing of shoes, especially after exercising, the feet should be washed with water and dried. Care should be taken to dry the area between the toes and keep them dry. (See Foot Care in *Diabetic Foot* -Book 1).

- One should not walk outdoors with bare feet and in water soaked areas. Footwear should be worn when possible. People working or walking in fields should preferably wear long rubber boots (gum boots).

- Avoiding close contact with animals as far as possible is advised for the elderly. Contact with animals having untreated skin infections should be avoided.

- Care should be taken to dry oneself well with a dry towel after bathing or swimming. The area between the toes, groins and below the breasts in women should be cleaned.

Fungal infection of Nail (Tinea Unguium)

The nails of the hands or feet may be affected. The fungus infects and grows in the nail or under the nail. It can spread from person to person. Use of infected instruments while doing manicure or pedicure or using the nail cutter of person who has infected nails, may transmit it to others. The persons at risk of developing fungal infection of the nail are:

- Diabetics and other immunocompromised persons.
- Those who have nail injury or bite their nails.
- When fingers or toes are exposed to moisture and wetness for long periods as in housewives who wash dishes or wash clothes by hand, washermen, farmers who work barefoot in the field.
- Use of a common swimming pool or those who swim in ponds

and other closed water bodies.

- Persons using artificial nails.
- Those who wear shoes for long periods especially in hot humid climates.
- Those elderly with poor circulation in the legs due to diseases of the arteries of the lower limb.
- Those above the age of 65.

Symptoms of fungal infection of the nail are seen as thickening of the nail and discoloration. The nail assumes a whitish or yellowish color with patches or streaks in it. Often the nail lifts off from the nail bed and becomes distorted, brittle, and breaks off easily. The skin at the base of the nail may be red and swollen.

Treatment. The treatment of the fungal infection is often prolonged and should be done on the advice of a physician or Dermatologist. The nail may have to be removed surgically in some individuals. In others, a medicated solution may be applied to the nails. Severe infections need oral medications to be taken for long periods of time, often months.

Prevention. Preventing nail infections becomes very important in those patients who are old or have risk factors. Some of the tips for preventing fungal infections of the nails are:

- Care should be taken not to injure or damage the skin at the base of the nails (cuticle).
- Prolonged exposure of hands to water must be avoided. If one has to work with wet hands for long periods, gloves must be worn to prevent fungal infection.
- The feet should be dried well after bathing and the area between the toes should be properly dried.
- Walking barefoot outdoors, in fields and on wet ground should be avoided as far as possible.
- It is preferable to avoid using artificial nails and nail polish.

Having a pedicure or manicure should be from authorized salons where the instruments are properly sterilized before use.

Oral Thrush (Oral Candidiasis)

Oral Thrush is a condition where creamy-white patches occur in the lining of the mouth and tongue. In severe cases it can spread to the throat, roof of the mouth, and affect the *esophagus* to produce severe symptoms. It is common in infants and also in elderly persons with reduced immunity. Our mouth normally contains the fungus called *Candida albicans*. It is often present in the skin, gut, and the vagina. This fungus causes no problem in normal individuals. But in conditions where immunity is lowered as in cancers, AIDS, and other immunosuppressed conditions, the fungus overgrows to produce these patches.

What are the symptoms of Oral Thrush

- The person feels sore in the mouth and a burning sensation which causes difficulty in eating and swallowing.
- The creamy white patches which look like flakes of cheese are seen in the mouth and throat.
- These lesions may bleed when scraped.
- The corners of the mouth may be cracked and red.
- The individual with candidiasis may experience a cotton-like feeling in the mouth.
- There may be loss of taste in the person with oral thrush.
- When it affects the esophagus, the patient feels pain when swallowing solids.

Candidiasis of the mouth and esophagus can occur in the following conditions.

- Diabetes, especially if it is uncontrolled and the blood sugars are very high.

- Immunosuppressed conditions like HIV/AIDS and organ transplanted individuals.
- Those who are on antibiotics or steroid medications for long periods.
- Cancer, especially when treated with chemotherapy or radiation.
- Smokers, those who wear dentures and patients who have a dry mouth due to any cause are liable to develop oral thrush.
- The fungal infection can also affect the vagina in females causing pain during sexual intercourse, burning sensation in the vagina and a bad-smelling fluid oozing out from the vagina.

Oral and vaginal thrush can be transmitted to the partner by kissing and sexual intercourse.

The disease can be easily diagnosed by the doctor on clinical examination. A scraping from the white patch can be examined under the microscope in a laboratory to identify the fungus. Tests like *esophagoscopy* may be needed to diagnose thrush in the esophagus.

How is the disease treated.

The disease in the mouth and throat can be treated with anti-fungal medications. They are available as mouth washes which can be rinsed around in the mouth and gargled. Lozenges are also available which can be sucked for mild infections in the mouth and throat. In severe cases affecting the esophagus, oral medications or injections may be needed. Vaginal candidiasis may be treated with vaginal applications of the medications in the form of vaginal creams or *suppositories*.

How can candidiasis be prevented.

The main points in the prevention of candidiasis are as follows:

- Cleanliness and hygiene are the two main factors needed in prevention. Whenever steroid inhalers are used, the mouth should be rinsed with water to remove any residual medication in the mouth or throat.

- The elderly should take care to brush their teeth twice a day.
- Those who wear dentures should keep them clean. Dentures should be removed at night and placed in water. The dentures should fit well. Cleaning agents for dentures are available and may be used on the advice of the dental surgeon.
- Dry mouth should be treated by a doctor depending on the cause.
- Sugary substances can cause oral thrush. It is better to limit the intake of sweets.
- Diabetics should be careful to keep their blood sugar under control.
- Women should keep the genitals clean and wear cotton underclothes. Any suspicion of vaginal thrush should be immediately treated.
- Sharing cups, spoons or forks with others may transmit the disease and should be avoided.

VIRAL INFECTIONS

Of the few important viral infections of the skin that can affect the elderly population, *Herpes Zoster* is the most important. Other viral diseases affecting the elderly are *Herpes Simplex* and *Molluscum Contagiosum*.

Herpes Zoster.

It is also called 'Shingles'. It is a disease seen in the skin in the elderly usually after the age of 50. Chicken pox (Varicella) is a disease commonly seen in children where it may not be serious in most of them. Following an infection with Chicken pox virus in young age, the virus remains inactive in the nerves arising from the spinal cord. Later in life when the individual's immunity wanes, it appears in the form of skin infection as Herpes Zoster or Shingles.

The lifetime risk of developing the disease is 20-30% and after the age of 80 it may be up to 50%. In the USA approximately one million people contract the disease yearly.

The virus which lies inactive in the nerves of the spinal cord after an attack of Chicken pox gets activated when the person grows old or develops an immunocompromised state like cancer, AIDS, treatment with immunosuppressant medications as for organ transplantation, or bone marrow transplantation.

What are the symptoms of Herpes zoster.

- Initially, a burning or tingling sensation may occur in the skin in a part of the body. The whole body is not involved as in Chicken pox. The area of skin involved corresponds to the area which the infected nerve supplies. Occasionally it may occur in the face when one of the nerves arising from the brain supplying the face is involved. The burning pain may precede the development of the rash by many days.
- The rashes appear next. They are seen as itchy fluid filled blisters. The skin is red and there is associated intense pain. The skin is painful to touch.
- The rash appears in a band or belt-like fashion on the body which corresponds to the nerve supply to that area.
- Some patients experience fever and headache along with the appearance of the rashes. Severe tiredness is noticed in some.
- The blisters dry up and form crusts and usually it takes two to four weeks for the blisters to disappear. Occasionally they leave scars or a dark pigmentation.

The elderly may be immunocompromised and hence the disease may be more severe in them. The complications of the disease are also more in the elderly individuals compared to young adults.

What are complications of Herpes zoster

- Neuralgia or severe pain in the area of distribution of the affected nerve may continue for weeks or months after the rashes have healed and rarely for years in some patients. This is called *Post Herpetic Neuralgia*. The older the individual, the greater the chances of developing this complication.
- Elderly patients with Herpes zoster run the risk of developing **Heart attack** or **Stroke** in the six months following the infection. The chance of stroke is increased when the face is involved.
- Rarely Herpes zoster may affect the eye and cause scarring and **loss of vision**. This is a very dangerous situation.
- Shingles also has been found to increase the risk of developing **dementia** as it may involve the smaller blood vessels of the brain.
- In a very small fraction of cases (<1%) it can lead to **death**.
- The *vesicles* may get infected by bacteria like Staphylococcus and produce serious **bacterial infection**, which on healing can leave scars.
- Occasionally, shingles can cause **paralysis of muscles** especially of the face and other muscles in the body supplied by the affected nerve. When the nerve to the ear is affected, **deafness** may occur.
- Rarely, Herpes zoster may affect the brain to cause inflammation in the brain (*Encephalitis*) which can be fatal.
- Some elderly patients develop mental depression after an attack of shingles.

Though shingles is not directly infectious to others, the vesicles are filled with fluid which contain the virus. This virus can infect others if they have not been vaccinated or did not have Chicken pox in the past and cause infection (Chicken pox) in them. Hence unvaccinated children should not be exposed to elders with shingles.

How is Shingles treated.

- Even though the disease subsides spontaneously in 2 – 4 weeks in untreated individuals, the disease must be treated promptly to prevent complications and extension of the disease.
- Anti-viral medications are prescribed for the disease and should be taken 3 – 5 times a day depending on the type of medication prescribed. Most of these drugs are given for seven days.
- Simple pain medications may suffice in most patients but some require stronger medications for relief of the pain. Soothing applications of Calamine lotion are helpful in early stages.
- Steroids are given in some patients to reduce the inflammation due to the disease and when the brain is involved as in encephalitis.
- Post Herpetic Neuralgia needs more intensive treatment. Opium-like medications, anti-epilepsy medications or anti-depressants may be needed in severe nerve pain. Occasionally anesthetic ointments applied to the area give pain relief. In severe cases of Neuralgia, the nerve supplying to the area is blocked by injection of an anesthetic medication into the nerve.
- Interestingly, one study has shown that mindfulness meditation is of benefit in relieving the pain of Herpes zoster.
- When the eye is involved, an Ophthalmologist must be consulted and appropriate treatment given to prevent scarring and loss of vision.

Prevention. The main aspect of prevention is vaccination. The elderly above the age of 50 should be vaccinated against Herpes zoster. Two injections 2 to 6 months apart are given as recommended by the Advisory Committee on Immunization Practices.

Herpes Simplex

Herpes simplex virus (**HSV**) causes skin lesions which are painful and itchy. There are two types of this virus – HSV-1 and HSV-2. HSV-1 causes skin lesions around the mouth and can spread through saliva. Whereas HSV-2 produces lesion in the genitals and is sexually transmitted causing sores in the genitals of the sexual partner.

It is estimated that about 3.7 billion persons below the age of 50, globally have HSV-1 infection.(*W.H.O.*). Herpes simplex virus can be transmitted to a child when adults with the virus their saliva kiss the child. Majority of healthy individuals already harbor the virus but owing to their strong immunity, they do not show any symptoms. During conditions like high fever or situations when the immunity is reduced, they develop sores around the mouth in the margins of the lips (*Cold sore*). These can occur recurrently.

HSV-1 can be transmitted from person to person by kissing, sharing utensils like spoons or cups, lip balms or lipstick, shaving razors, or coming in contact with the saliva of a person infected with the virus. Once the virus is acquired, it remains inactive within the nerves of the person.. It flares up during periods when the person's immunity is low like fever, stress, or immunosuppressed conditions in old age.

HSV-2 can be transmitted from person to person during sexual intercourse or intimate contact. Contact with the sores in the genitals or breast can transmit the disease. It is estimated that 491 million people between the ages of 1- and 49 have HSV-2 infection globally.(WHO).

Symptoms.

HSV-1 infection can be *asymptomatic* or present as sores around the mouth at the margins of the lips. In some they can be seen as painful ulcers around the mouth and lips. They subside spontaneously in most patients. The patient feels a burning sensation around the mouth. Sometimes the patient can develop fever and enlargement of the lymph nodes along with the fever and sores. These disappear once the fever subsides and may reappear at a later time.

HSV-2 infection can produce itchy blisters around the genitals – penis in the male and vagina in the female. They may also occur around the anus. These usually break down to produce oozing lesions. Occasionally the patient develops mild fever, muscle pains, swelling of lymph nodes and tiredness. This may last from two to four weeks.

Rarely in the elderly and immunocompromised individuals, HSV infection can affect the brain to cause brain infection (*encephalitis*) and infection in the eye.

The HSV infection can be diagnosed by a blood test and also by examining a swab from the oozing lesions.

Treatment of Herpes Simplex Virus Infection.

There is no total cure for Herpes simplex infection. The virus persists in the body, but the symptoms clear away by themselves even without treatment. But often treatment is initiated because, it can cut short the clinical course of the disease. An antiviral cream relieves the itching and burning sensation. Anti-viral medications can be given orally or as injections to cut short the illness. The first infection with the virus is usually of fairly severe nature whereas the subsequent recurrences are not that severe. The first outbreak of genital herpes lasts for about two to four weeks whereas repeated outbreaks last only for less than a week.

Applying ice packs to the blisters may reduce the soreness and the burning sensation. If there is pain, tablets for pain may be given. Tight clothes should not be worn. The area should be kept clean and dry.

It is to be noted that persons with HSV-2 infection are more likely to contract HIV infection compared to normal people. The risk is said to be three times normal. Severe brain infection (*Encephalitis*) can occur in the immunocompromised people and the elderly.

How can HSV infection be prevented.

People with oral herpes should avoid close contact with others like kissing or using items like cups and spoons used by them. Saliva of persons with open ulcers is infective and hence care should be taken to keep away from them. Hand washing should be done frequently when handling these patients.

Persons with open genital ulceration should avoid sex during the active stage of the disease. Later they should use condoms while having sex. They should avoid having multiple sexual partners.

Medical circumcision can give some protection against HSV-2 though this is not absolute.

Molluscum Contagiosum

Molluscum contagiosum (**MC**) is a viral infection which can be seen in children and adults. Elderly and the immunocompromised individuals may contract the disease by spread from children in the home. It is spread by skin to skin contact. It tends to occur more in warm humid climates. Overcrowding is also a cause for spread of this infection. The disease can be spread by contact with infected objects. Children can acquire the disease from school. Adults can get during sexual contact or close contact with those infected.

The skin lesions are seen on the face, neck, arms, body, and hands. They are seen as rounded small pearl-like swellings with a central dimple. They vary in size from 1 mm to 5-7 mm in size. On pressing them a cheesy material is expelled which teems with viruses and is highly infective.

What are the symptoms of MC.

The infection starts as a tiny swelling on the skin which gradually enlarges in size. It does not grow to very big size. Itching may spread the infection to the adjacent parts of the skin or to other parts of the body in the same individual. They are painless but may be itchy. The tendency to scratch the itchy lesions may introduce bacteria into them causing bacterial infection.

How are they treated.

Often they disappear spontaneously in a period of 6 – 9 months but may need to be treated if they are present in large numbers or if the patient is immunocompromised.

Molluscum can be treated in various ways. But it is safer to get the opinion of a doctor to treat them. Self-medication should not be attempted.

- They can be removed with a needle by scraping them after sterilizing the area. This is called *Curettage*.
- They can be frozen with liquid nitrogen. This is called *Cryotherapy*.
- Wart removing plasters or creams also may be used.

How can MC be prevented.

- Hand washing is one of the best methods to avoid the disease.
- The small swellings should not be touched as they can spread the virus.
- Personal items like razors, brushes, makeup items and towels should not be shared by others as these can spread the virus.
- As they can be spread by sexual contact, sexual contact with persons with the disease must be avoided.
- When they are few in number, they can be covered with a plaster to avoid spreading the virus to others accidentally.

PARASITIC INFESTATIONS

The word '*Infestation*' refers to a condition where parasites like ticks, mites or insects live in the human body either on the skin or inside the body as in intestinal worms Skin *infestation* with parasites is not uncommon in the elderly especially in those who live in nursing homes and institutions. The two most common infestations are Scabies and Pediculosis or head lice. In the elderly, diagnosis may be difficult as the symptoms may not be typical as in the young and the presence of other diseases may deter an early diagnosis. Furthermore, the additional presence of immunosuppression, and mental or physical disability in these patients may render them easily susceptible to these infestations.

Scabies

Scabies is caused by a parasite named *Sarcoptes scabiei* or *Itch Mite*. It spreads by close contact with other infested persons in crowded places like nursing homes, prisons, camps, families, and schools. It can also be spread by sharing personal items like towels, bedding, pillows, and other objects. The elderly are a vulnerable group for the spread of the infestation. The mite burrows into the skin and lays eggs. They produce tiny, raised lesions or blisters.

What are the symptoms of Scabies.

The typical symptoms are

- Intense itching is the chief symptom and is worse at night. The itching is due to allergy to the mite, its *feces,* and eggs.
- The disease affects the wrists, axilla, groin, buttocks, area around the umbilicus and nipple, genitalia, webs between the fingers of the hands and the thighs.
- In the elderly patient, scabies may have a different presentation. They may have the lesions on the face and soles of the feet unlike the younger population.
- Elderly patients who have cognitive impairment or loss of

memory may not be aware of the infestation and hence the disease spreads and becomes more severe in them. This is seen more in mental health institutions. In addition, the poor immune system and nutritional deficiencies in the elderly may predispose to severe infestation.

- The elderly may develop thickened crusts due to the disease called '*Crusted Scabies*' or '*Norwegian Scabies*'. These crusts contain thousands of mites and are highly contagious.

The disease is diagnosed by observing the skin with a magnifying glass. The physician or Dermatologist is able to recognize the irregular burrows in the skin caused by the mite. Scrapings from the skin are examined under the microscope and they show the typical mite and their eggs.

How is Scabies treated in the elderly.

Treatment consists in eradication of the mites from the skin of the patient. All the family members should be treated simultaneously as the others are also likely to be affected.

- A *scabicide*, Permethrin is used to treat scabies. It is available as a cream or lotion applied all over the body from head to foot taking care to avoid the eyes. It is left in place for 12-14 hours and washed away. Most patients get over the infestation with one application, but in severe infestations, a repeat application after two weeks may become necessary.
- Orally administered medication is available. It is given as two doses a week or two apart.
- Other applications containing sulfur, benzyl benzoate and other medications are available for the treatment of scabies. These are used in many developing countries as they are low-cost medications and may be needed in crowded conditions like camps, slums etc.
- In Crusted scabies, the application of Permethrin should be

done daily for a week followed by repeated applications at weekly intervals till the infestation clears completely. This is often combined with oral medicine.

- Itching may persist for a few days after treatment and may be controlled with anti-allergy tablets.

Prevention of Scabies.

Personal hygiene is most important in preventing the infestations. The elderly at home may contract the disease when children at home bring the infestation from school and spread it among the family members.

Washing the clothes in hot water and drying them in the sun are simple measures adopted in many tropical countries. Hot wash and dryers may be used in washing machines. Ironing the clothes, especially the innerwear helps destroy any mites that may be present in the clothes.

All family members must be examined for the disease, if one member has the infestation.

Special care must be taken in institutions and nursing homes housing the elderly. Any itching in an elderly patient must be checked immediately.

Pediculosis

Lice infestation is called *Pediculosis*. Different types of lice can affect different parts of the body. The common sites are head and the body. The chances of infestation are more in crowded living as in nursing homes, refugee camps, orphanages, shelters for the destitute and institutions for the elderly. Mental health facilities are places where lice infestation can occur and spread from person to person.

The lice are tiny insects which live on the surface of the human body and feed on blood. A different type of lice infest the pubic hair. This type is called the *'crab louse'* as it looks like a crab under the microscope. This is transmitted by sexual contact in most persons.

What are the symptoms of infestation with lice.

Though the symptoms are similar, they are described separately for convenience.

Head lice

- Itching of the scalp is the characteristic feature. Itching increases at night as the lice feed on blood from the scalp at night.
- The patient has red rashes and sores on the scalp.
- They may feel a crawling sensation in the scalp due to the live lice.
- The lice are visible to the naked eye on the scalp.
- Whitish dot like structures are seen attached to the hair of the scalp. They are the eggs of the lice and are called *Nits*.

Body lice

- This presents as itching of the infested region of the body like the pubic area, groin, and thighs.
- The itching can cause open ulcers and may get infected with bacteria.
- The patient feels a crawling sensation at the site and live lice can be seen crawling on the skin.
- The crab lice in the pubic area are seen attached to the hair.
- Intense itching can leave crusts due to clotted blood in elderly individuals who have sensitive skins.

Body lice can spread certain diseases like Relapsing fever and Typhus; hence they must be treated at the earliest. The complications of body lice are secondary bacterial infection occurring due to constant scratching, thickening and discoloration of the skin due to prolonged, untreated infestation.

How is Lice infestation treated.

The main aspects of treating lice infestation are removing the infesting insects and preventing recurrence. In a community infection, the whole group of patients should be treated simultaneously.

- For treating head lice, medicated shampoos with Pyrethrin or Permethrin are applied to the scalp, rubbed in, and allowed to remain for some time and washed off. *Care should be taken to prevent the medication from entering the eyes.* If they enter the eyes, the eyes should be washed with plenty of water immediately.
- Oral medications may be needed in heavy infestations and resistant cases.
- Itching may be relieved with anti-allergic medications.
- Soothing applications like calamine may be applied to the skin to lessen the irritation.
- To treat body lice, lotions containing the medication can be applied to the body.
- The hair should be combed with a fine toothed comb to remove the nits and dead lice after the application of medication. Whenever possible, removal of hair is advised. It makes treatment easier. All infested inmates in a facility should be simultaneously treated.
- Retreatment may be needed in severe infestation after 7-10 days when the remaining lice and those which hatched after the initial treatment are killed.
- Many of the medications for treatment of head lice are available over the counter (OTC). But the instructions on the label should be strictly followed while using them.

Prevention of lice infestation.

- Avoiding contact with persons infested with the lice.
- Sharing clothing or bedding with them should be avoided.

- Clothes and bed linen should be washed in hot water and machine dried or dried in the sun. The sun's rays are the best 'disinfectant' for the lice.
- Sharing of combs, brushes, towels, head bands, and toiletries should be avoided. Combs and brushes used by infested persons should be put in boiling water for 10-15 minutes.

ECZEMA

This is also called *Atopic Dermatitis* in medical parlance. The condition indicates various types of skin swelling. Eczema is a condition where there is swelling with blister formation, itching and occasionally bleeding. It can occur due to various causes. Eczema occurs in the elderly too. Seen more during winter, it is due to the cold, wind, the sun, and low humidity. Even though the commonest site affected are the shins, this can occur in the thighs, back and abdomen also.

Asteatotic Eczema

This is a type of eczema occurring in the elderly due to drying of the skin. It is also called *"Winter Eczema"*. There are thick patches of dry skin with cracking and clefts in the skin. The skin becomes dry and scaly resembling a dried paddy field in summer with cracks in the mud. The skin is itchy and reddish or brown in color.

Treatment.

Emollients are substances that soften and soothe the skin. Substances like Petrolatum, Lanolin, Mineral oil and Dimethicone are emollients. They keep the skin moisturized.

Eczema can be prevented by the following measures:

- Do not expose the person to direct heat like a fireplace, warmer or room heater. Sitting close to the source of heat should be avoided.
- Do not bathe in hot water, lukewarm water should be preferred and is ideal in winter. Bathing should be limited to 5-7 minutes only.
- Harsh soaps should be avoided. Moisturizing soaps may be used. After bathing one should not towel vigorously. Soap substitutes may be used.
- An emollient cream must be applied to the body after drying.
- Using a humidifier in the room is preferable. If not available, a

basin of water in the room helps to keep the air moist.

- In resistant cases, a steroid cream may be applied in consultation with a Dermatologist.
- Stress is often present in these individuals and can aggravate the eczema and hence its management is important.
- In countries like India, bathing after an oil massage is an effective way of preventing dry skin. (See section on *Dry Skin*).

Other causes of eczema are Allergies, contact with certain metals, certain types of clothing like wool or polyester clothing, household detergents, perfumes, plants, and hair dye. It is wise to identify these triggers and eliminate them.

MISCELLANEOUS CONDITIONS

Management of Skin disorders in the Elderly

The management of skin disorders in the elderly population may pose challenges unlike those in young adults and children. Often the elderly may be physically or mentally challenged with problems like cognitive impairment or dementia and may not be able to take care of themselves. They may be dependent on others like their relatives or caregivers. They may be on multiple medications due to other systemic diseases which may cause skin reactions.

Many of the elders may be undernourished due to their independent living conditions. The elderly may be financially challenged and resort to treatment with over the counter medications or alternative medical treatments. Their living conditions too may not be ideal especially in winter and they may not be able to follow the medical advice given to them.

Some of the less common skin conditions seen in the elderly are given below.

Skin tags are common in old age. A skin tag is a piece of soft hanging skin with a stalk. They are harmless, *benign* (not cancerous) and often seen in significant numbers. They vary in size from 1 – 4 mm and occur in the neck, groin, and the armpit where there are skin folds. They are harmless, but for their cosmetic appearance. They can be removed by the Dermatologist. Diabetics and obese persons tend to have more skin tags. The individual should be advised not to remove the tag by themselves as it may cause severe bleeding.

Cherry Angiomas are seen in the elderly over the body and upper limbs. They are seen as red or purplish spots or tiny swellings and vary in size from 1 – 4 mm. they are harmless and more of cosmetic concern. After the age of 75 about three-fourth of the elders have these spots on their bodies. They need not be treated and may be left alone. They may be removed by the surgeon if they are of cosmetic concern.

Skin Cancers in the elderly can occur occasionally. Three types of skin cancers may occur. They are Basal Cell Carcinoma, Squamous Cell Carcinoma and Melanoma. This classification is based on the microscopic type of cell seen in the cancer. Skin cancers can occur in areas exposed to sunlight when the person is young. But they may also occur in areas not exposed to sunlight. Melanoma is the cancer which is most aggressive and often fatal. They spread rapidly.

Melanomas arise from the pigment cells in the skin (*Melanocyte*). The risk factors for developing melanoma are cited as follows:

- Those with very fair skin.
- Excess exposure to sunlight.
- History of melanoma in the family members.
- Presence of large moles in the body or an unusual number of moles.
- Blue-eyed individuals and those with red or blond hair are also said to be at a higher risk of melanoma.

Those who have large moles or moles with an irregular edge or a sudden enlargement of size in a mole should be brought to the attention of the doctor for further evaluation. Various methods of treatment are available and the dermatologist will give appropriate advice on the type of treatment to be followed.

Nutritional disorders of skin are also not uncommon in the elderly population. Women, especially of advanced age tend to suffer from nutritional deficiencies of vitamins B 12, C, D, and minerals like iron, zinc, calcium, and others. These may cause changes in the skin and may be mistaken for primary disease of the skin. It is mandatory for the elderly to have a balanced nutritious diet and in some cases, a vitamin-mineral supplementation may be needed.

Resources

1. Gerontodermatology: The fragility of the Epidermis in older Adults:

Katoh N et al. *Journal of European Academy of Dermatology & Venereology.* 2018, 32 (Suppl 4) pages 1 – 20.

2. Geriatric Dermatoses: A clinical Review of Skin Diseases in an Aging population. Jafferany M et al. *International Journal of Dermatology.* 2012. 51 Pages 509-522.

3. Geriatric Dermatology: A Framework for Caring for Older patients with Skin Disease. Linos E et al. *JAMA Dermatology* – 2018.

4. Xerosis: Symptoms, Causes and Treatment Tips. – *Curel*

https://www.curel.com/en-us/dry-skin/xerosis/

1. Dry Skin in the Elderly : *Senior Health 365*

https://www.seniorhealth365.com/health/dry-skin-in-the-elderly/

1. Pressure Ulcers : Overview. *National Health Service . UK.* 2020

https://www.nhs.uk/conditions/pressure-sores/

1. Treatment of pressure ulcers: a clinical practice guideline from the American College of Physicians. Qaseem A.et al. *Annals of Internal Medicine.* 2015. 162 : pages 370-379

https://pubmed.ncbi.nlm.nih.gov/25732279/

1. Types of Fungal Infections & Treatment Options : *Healthline*

https://www.healthline.com/health/fungal-skin-infection#risk-factors

1. Candida infections of the Mouth, Throat and Esophagus. *Centers for Disease Control and Prevention.*

https://www.cdc.gov/fungal/diseases/candidiasis/thrush/index.html

1. Herpes Zoster in Older Adults. Yoshikawa TT & Schmader K. *Clinical Infectious Disease.* 2001. Vol 32 pages 1481-1486.

https://academic.oup.com/cid/article/32/10/1481/467091

1. Shingles (Herpes Zoster) – Clinical Overview. *Centers for Disease Control & Prevention.* 2020

https://www.cdc.gov/shingles/hcp/
clinical-overview.html#:~:text=A%20person's%20risk%20of%20having,younger%20tha [1].

1. Skin Disorders in Elderly Persons: Identifying Viral Infections. Scheinfeld NS. *Infect Med.* 2007 24: 479 -481.

http://www.antimicrobe.org/h04c.files/history/
IIM-Skin%20Disorders%20in%20elderly%20persons-identifying%20viral%20infections

1. Herpes simplex : Diagnosis & Treatment. *American Academy of Dermatology.* 2022.

https://www.aad.org/public/diseases/a-z/herpes-simplex-treatment

1. Herpes Simplex Virus : Health Topics. *World Health Organization* 2022.

https://www.who.int/news-room/fact-sheets/detail/herpes-simplex-virus

1. Review of Scabies in the Elderly. Raffi J et al. *Dermatology & Therapy.* 2019. 9 : 623-630.

https://www.ncbi.nlm.nih.gov/pmc/articles/PMC6828878/

1. Parasites – Lice . *Centers for Disease Control & Prevention.*

---

1. https://www.cdc.gov/shingles/hcp/
clinical-overview.html#_853ae90f0351324bd73ea615e6487517__4c761f170e016836ff84498202b99827__853ae
90f0351324bd73ea615e6487517_text_43ec3e5dee6e706af7766fffea512721_A_0bcef9c45bd8a48eda1b26eb0c61
c869_20person_3590cb8af0bbb9e78c343b52b93773c9_s_0bcef9c45bd8a48eda1b26eb0c61c869_20risk_0bcef9c
45bd8a48eda1b26eb0c61c869_20of_0bcef9c45bd8a48eda1b26eb0c61c869_20having_c0cb5f0fcf239ab3d9c1fcd
31fff1efc_younger_0bcef9c45bd8a48eda1b26eb0c61c869_20than_0bcef9c45bd8a48eda1b26eb0c61c869_2040_
0bcef9c45bd8a48eda1b26eb0c61c869_20years_0bcef9c45bd8a48eda1b26eb0c61c869_20old

https://www.cdc.gov/parasites/lice/index.html

1. Head and Body Lice in the Elderly. *Senior Health 365*. Nov 2022.

https://www.seniorhealth365.com/health/head-and-body-lice-in-the-elderly/

3. THE EYE

The eye is the organ of sight in an organism. The human eye ball is situated safely in a socket formed by a fusion of many bones in the skull. This socket is called the *Orbit*. It is about one inch (22-24mm) in diameter. At the back of this socket is a small hole through which the nerve of the eye called the *Optic nerve* exits to join the brain.

The eyelids which are made of skin, thin sheet of muscle and an inner transparent membrane called *Conjunctiva* protect the eye from injury. They help to spread the tears secreted by the tear glands situated in the sides of the eyes uniformly so as to prevent drying of the eyes. This happens when we blink. A normal person blinks every 2-10 seconds.

The eye is able to see nearly 200 degrees in all directions. It is able to recognize thousands of shades of color. Both the eyes work in a coordinated manner to give a three dimensional (stereoscopic) effect to the images that we see.

The **Conjunctiva** is a thin transparent membrane which covers the inner aspect of the eyelids and the front of the eye which is white in color – the Sclera.

The **Sclera** is the white portion of the eyeball that we see surrounding the central Iris.

The **Iris** is the rounded colored part of the eye seen in the center. It has various shades of color in different individuals. the iris is a ring shaped curtain which can alter the amount of light entering the eye. The central dark rounded opening at the center of the iris is called the **Pupil**. The Iris can decrease or increase the size of the pupil when it is bright or dark respectively to regulate the amount of light entering the eye. The iris may be blue, brown, gray, hazel, green or have other shades of color.

The **Cornea** is the clear window-like transparent part of the eye which covers the front of the eye and permits light to enter the eye.

The **Lens** of the eye is in the center behind the iris. It is biconvex in shape, transparent and is a semi-solid structure capable of changing shape mildly due to thin ring-shaped muscles which control it from the sides. These are called **Ciliary muscles** and they help to change the shape of the lens to adjust for near and distant vision by focusing the light on the retina. (**Figure 3**)

The **Retina** is the 'screen' at the back of the eyeball on which the images we see fall. It is composed of two types of cells called the Rods and Cones. The rods help us to see in dim light and the cones help us see in bright light and identify colors.

The **Macula** is a group of cells in the area at the back of eye in the retina. This helps in giving us a clear, sharp image of objects and their finer details in the center of the field of vision.

The **Vitreous** is a transparent jelly-like substance which fills the eyeball behind the lens.

The **Optic Nerve** is a thick nerve which arises from the back of the retina and exits through the small hole at the back of the Orbit to join the brain. It contains about one million nerve fibers. It carries the signals from the retina to the brain where it is interpreted into images which we see.

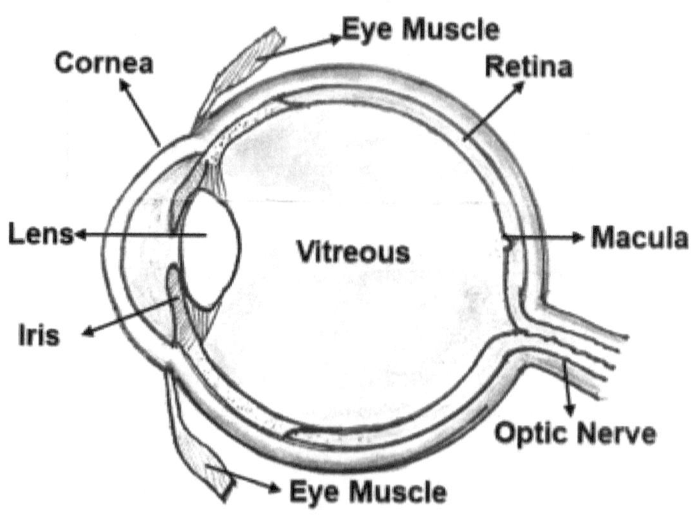

Figure 3

The part of the eye behind the cornea and in front of the lens is filled with a transparent fluid called **Aqueous Humor**. This fluid nourishes the lens because there are no blood vessels in the lens to supply nutrients as in other parts of the body.

There are six small ribbon-like muscles attached to the sides of the eye. They are attached to the bone at the back of the orbit. They help to move the eye in all directions. In addition, a seventh thin muscle is attached to the upper eyelid and helps to elevate (open) the eyelid.

The eye functions like a camera. The light from the external object falls on the lens of the eye. The lens converges this light to fall on the retina. The cells in the retina convert this light energy to electrical energy or signals which are transmitted to the brain through the optic nerve. The brain interprets these signals as visual images.

The amount of light entering the eye is controlled by the iris which alters the size of the pupil. In bright light, the pupil becomes very small and in dim light the pupil enlarges in size to permit more light to enter the eye.

The **Tear glands** on the outer sides of the eyes secrete tears which are produced continuously to keep the front of the eye and the cornea moist. The tears contain water and electrolytes and an enzyme which can destroy bacteria to some extent. Any irritation to the eye like a foreign body or irritant can induce a copious secretion of tears which flushes away the irritant. Tears are also secreted by stimulation of the tongue by spices, inner lining of the nose by irritant odor or infections and by emotion.

The elderly population in the United States is increasing. By the year 2030, it is estimated that there will be 70 million people above the age of 65. The eye is one of the most important sense organs that invariably undergoes changes in old age. One of the main problems associated with old age is the impairment of vision.

It was found that in a Nursing home in Delaware, 63.8% of the subjects above the age of 65 living there were visually impaired or blind. Cataract was present in 60% of the inmates, 75% had macular degeneration, 26% had glaucoma and 7.75 had Diabetic retinopathy. This in brief summarizes the four common problems encountered in old age. Other problems noted are presbyopia and dry eyes.

As a person ages, his *visual acuity* becomes weaker. It is important to know what to expect when one grows old and when to seek medical professional help. Some of the conditions of the eye in the elderly are painless and slow in onset, and hence, the person may be totally unaware of the changes occurring in his eye. In addition, other medical illnesses too may cause changes in the eye.. The seriousness of these conditions vary. Some of these conditions are discussed below.

PRESBYOPIA

By the age of 40, an individual begins to lose the ability to see small print or objects close to the eye clearly. When they read, they may have to hold the books at arm's length. This is associated with tiredness of the eyes and occasionally headache. It is due to the inability of the eyes to focus on nearby objects and is called *Presbyopia*. It means "Old Eye" in Greek. Normally in the young, the eye can see objects which are near and far by a process called '*Accommodation*'. The lens of the eye changes shape slightly to see the near and far away objects because of its soft and elastic nature. But as age advances, the lens of the eye becomes more rigid and the ability to change shape or 'accommodate' decreases. The persons finds it difficult to read small print and see objects close to the eye like threading a needle or sewing.

What are the symptoms of Presbyopia.

The symptoms of Presbyopia start around the age of 40. The commonest symptom of Presbyopia is the inability to read at the normal distance and view objects closer to the eye. The distant objects are however seen clearly. This may be accompanied by eye strain and fatigue. Often the person needs bright light when reading or doing any work related to near objects like stitching, repairing small objects, etc. They would have to hold objects at arm's length to see them clearly. Often squinting of the eyes is required to bring the objects or print into focus. This can lead to eye strain and headaches.

Risk factors for developing Presbyopia.

1. Age is the most important risk factor as presbyopia is inevitable in old age.

2. Diseases like Diabetes mellitus, and diseases of the heart and blood vessels can lead to premature presbyopia.

3. Certain medications like antidepressants and medications used for the treatment of allergies may cause premature presbyopia in some individuals.

4. Presbyopia may occur early after head injury.

5. Being 'far-sighted' or 'long-sighted' can lead to early development of presbyopia.

What can be done to correct Presbyopia.

1. Simple measures in early stages of the problem can be overcome by keeping the reading material a little away from the eyes for reading to avoid eye strain.
2. Increasing the brightness of light for reading or using table lamps in addition to the room lighting helps in early stages.
3. When the presbyopia is more advanced and causes symptoms like eye strain or headache, an *Ophthalmologist* should be consulted and corrective glasses prescribed. This is done after a simple test called *Optometry* where the appropriate lens is chosen for the individual to correct the visual disturbance. This can be worn as a spectacle or as contact lenses.
4. For those with presbyopia alone, reading glasses are enough. They can be worn during reading or performing near work to prevent strain on the eye. The exact power of the lens is determined by testing with various lenses.
5. Some individuals have both presbyopia and short-sightedness (*Myopia*). Various type of lenses are available for correcting this. The bifocal lenses are the commonest. The eyeglasses have two lenses. The one at the top corrects for distant vision and the lower one corrects the near vision or presbyopia. Other eyeglasses called 'Progressives' are available where there are multifocal lenses which show a gradual shift from distant

vision to near vision from top to bottom. Various types of contact lenses are available for correction of presbyopia.

6. Surgery is available today for the correction of presbyopia. This may be done on the advice of the eye surgeon. When cataract is present along with presbyopia, the Ophthalmologist removes the lens of the eye and substitutes an artificial lens implanted into the eye.

How can presbyopia be prevented.

Presbyopia is a part of the aging process and cannot be prevented. However, certain precautions can be taken to delay its onset and mitigate its effects.

- One should always use adequate lighting while reading or doing near work to prevent eyestrain.
- A healthy nutritious diet is important for eye health. One should include green leafy vegetables in the diet. Vitamin A is essential for eye health and it is available in vegetables like sweet potato, green leafy vegetables like spinach, kale, carrots, and red peppers. Vitamin A is available in fruits like mango, papaya, persimmon, watermelon, apricot and guava. Animal based foods like liver, fish and cheese also contain vitamin A. the daily requirement of Vitamin A is 900 mcg for men, 700 mcg for women and 300–600 mcg for children and adolescents. In addition, Vitamins C and E are also important for eye health.
- Smoking should be avoided. Alcohol intake should also be moderated.
- Regular exercise helps to keep the eyes healthy.
- Sunglasses should be worn whenever possible outdoors during summer to protect the eyes from the harmful ultraviolet rays of the sun.

- Diabetes and High blood pressure, if present should be controlled well with adequate medications and frequent visits to the doctor.

A yearly visit to the Ophthalmologist after the age of 40 is ideal to care for one's eye. The American Academy of Ophthalmology recommends that adults have a complete eye exam every:

⬦ Five to 10 years under age 40
⬦ Two to four years between ages 40 and 54
⬦ One to three years between ages 55 and 64
⬦ One to two years beginning at age 65

CATARACT

Literally, the word 'Cataract' means a 'Waterfall'. Medically, it is a condition where the lens of the eye becomes opaque gradually leading to visual impairment and total blindness. Cataract is an important cause of blindness in the world and is responsible for 40% of cases of blindness or visual impairment. In a healthy person, the lens of the eye is totally transparent permitting light to enter the eye normally. When a cataract occurs, the lens gradually becomes cloudy and ends up being opaque. Initially, cataract may start as a small patch in a part of the lens and as days go by, it enlarges to opacify the whole lens. Cataract is treatable by surgery which is available all over the world.

What are the symptoms of cataract.

The symptoms of cataract are gradual in onset and progressive in nature. They are:

- Gradual onset of blurring of vision.
- A tendency to squint the eye when in bright light or sunlight.
- The person may see halos around bright light and have difficulty in driving at night.
- Frequent squinting may lead to recurrent headaches.
- Colors may seem blurred.
- During the early stages of cataract, the person may see double. Often it is said that he sees two moons at night. Later this symptom may disappear as the cataract progresses.

What causes cataract.

Cataract usually is a disease of the elderly and is a part of aging. But there are other causes of cataract that may occur at any age and even at birth. Some of the causes of cataracts are as follows:

- Exposure to ultraviolet light as occurs in persons working in sunny climates and at high ranges.

- Physical injury to the eye can lead to cataract at any age.
- Cataract at birth may occur in babies occasionally due to genetic disorders of if the mother contracts Rubella ('German Measles') during pregnancy.
- Smoking can cause cataract early in life.
- Diabetes mellitus is a cause of premature cataract.
- Long term use of drugs like steroids can lead to cataracts.
- Exposure to ionizing radiation causes cataracts.

How is Cataract treated.

The treatment of cataract is surgical. There is no medical treatment for the condition. However, in early stages, some simple measures helps the person with cataract to improve his vision.

Having a bright light while reading and working with near objects, reading books with a large print, or using magnifying glasses, avoiding glare by using sunglasses outdoors are some of the measures one can adopt during the early stages.

Changing the power of one's eyeglasses may give better vision for some time, but surgery will be needed at a later date.

Surgery is done in advanced cases where there is a significant impairment of vision,. The Ophthalmologist will advise the type of surgery suitable for the person. During surgery, the opaque, damaged lens of the eye is removed and replaced with a transparent implantable artificial lens. This is called the *"Intra Ocular Lens"* (IOL).

Prevention of Cataract.

World over approximately 1 billion people have visual impairment. Low and middle income countries account for 90% of this population. Surprisingly, 90% of the visual loss can be prevented or treated. Even though there are no definite ways to prevent cataract, the following measures are helpful.

- A diet rich in vegetables and fruits along with animal foods like cheese, liver and fish helps in making adequate vitamins like A, C and E available which are important in eye health.

- Smoking is an avoidable risk factor for cataract and quitting smoking is very important.
- Wearing sunglasses reduces the risk of developing cataracts by cutting down the ultraviolet rays entering the eyes.
- Limiting alcohol intake is important in prevention.
- Diabetics should take care to keep their blood sugars under control.
- A yearly eye examination should be done after the age of 60.

GLAUCOMA

Glaucoma is a condition where the pressure inside the eyeball increases. The normal eyeball is filled with a clear fluid in its front part. It is called **Aqueous Humor** and is continuously produced and the excess fluid drained off. When the channel draining the fluid is blocked, the pressure inside the eyeball increases and this can lead to damage to the *Optic Nerve* causing poor vision and subsequent blindness.

The global prevalence of glaucoma is reported at 3.54%. It is estimated that by 2040 the number of cases of glaucoma globally will rise to 111.8 million. Approximately 3 million people in the USA are affected by glaucoma but only half of them are aware of it. Glaucoma is the cause of about 10% of the blindness in the USA.

What are the causes of glaucoma.

Some of the causes of glaucoma are:

- A Family history of glaucoma.
- Aging increases the chances of developing glaucoma. It is more common after the age of 60. Women are more prone to develop the disease.
- Injury to the eye can lead to glaucoma.
- Diabetes mellitus and High blood pressure.
- Long-sightedness.
- Short-sightedness.
- Ethnic background is important. African Americans are more prone to develop glaucoma between the ages of 40 an 80. The Japanese are more prone to develop glaucoma.
- Glaucoma may occur in a sleep disorder called Obstructive Sleep Apnea. (See section on *Obstructive Sleep Apnea* under *Sleep Disorders*).

What are the symptoms of glaucoma.

There are many different types of glaucoma. This depends on the cause and mechanism of the increase in pressure inside the eye. Some of the important symptoms of the disease are:

- In the early stages the patient may not have any symptoms. It develops slowly over many years with a gradual loss of vision.
- As the disease progresses, the patient develops pain in the eye and headache. The eye is often red and the pupil may be dilated (enlarged in size).
- Gradual loss of vision in the eye occurs involving the peripheral vision or side vision. Initially this may be a patchy loss of vision and later the side vision may be totally lost causing '*Tunnel Vision*' where the patient feels as if he is seeing through a tunnel or tube. Finally, the patient develops irreversible blindness.
- The patient may see rainbow colored rings (halos) around bright lights.
- Nausea and vomiting may occur when the pain in the eye is severe.

How is glaucoma treated.

There are many simple tests done by the Ophthalmologist to diagnose glaucoma. They are painless tests and measure the pressure inside the eyeball.

Initially, the treatment of the disease is with <u>eye drops</u> which help to drain the fluid from the eyeball and reduce the pressure within the eye.

<u>Medications</u> are given to ease the symptoms and promote drainage of fluid from the eye. In addition, diseases like diabetes and high blood pressure need to be strictly controlled.

<u>Surgery</u> is the final option in the treatment of glaucoma when medicines no longer give full relief to the patient. Different types of

the surgeries are available and the Ophthalmologist chooses the type of surgery that is optimal for the patient.

How can we prevent glaucoma.

- The most important approach to prevent the disease is to keep the risk factors like diabetes and high blood pressure well controlled with medications.
- A proper lifestyle of nutritious diet and adequate exercise helps.
- Reducing caffeine intake is found to be effective in prevention.
- Stress may precipitate an attack of acute glaucoma and hence stress management is important.
- Wearing protective eyewear while working in high risk jobs and during sports is necessary to prevent eye injuries which may lead to glaucoma.
- Regular yearly eye checkup is necessary after the age of 55 to assess the pressure inside the eyeball.
- Sudden onset of pain in the eye and headache may indicate acute glaucoma and is a medical emergency needing immediate care.

AGE RELATED MACULAR DEGENERATION

Age Related Macular Degeneration (**ARMD**) is a disease of the retina of the eye occurring in those over the age of 55 and is a common cause of loss of vision in the elderly.

The macula is that part of the *retina* which is at the center of the eyeball opposite the lens. It is the most sensitive part of the retina and is responsible for central vision. Damage to this part of the retina causes blurring of vision centrally leading to difficulty in seeing things right in front of the person. This makes it difficult for the individual to drive, read, cook, and recognize faces when looking forward directly. It usually does not cause total blindness but is highly disabling.

ARMD may be slow in onset in some, but in others the disease may progress rapidly. The global prevalence of ARMD was 196 million in 2020 and is expected to rise to 288 million by 2040, the maximum number of patients being in Asia.

What are the symptoms of ARMD.

The symptoms depend on the stage of the disease. The disease may be early, intermediate, or late. The symptoms are as follows:

- In the early stages of the disease the symptoms may be very minimal. Mild blurring of vision with reduced vision in dim light is often an early symptom.
- In later stages, the person may see straight lines as wavy.
- Central vision is impaired to a variable extent. In early stages, the blurring may be mild, but later the central area of visual defect increases in size.
- The individual may experience difficulty in distinguishing colors.
- The person complains that he is not able to recognize the faces of others.

- Driving becomes extremely difficult owing to the defect in central vision.
- In later stages of the disease, due to the deteriorating vision, the patient may go into mental depression.
- Some patients get visual hallucinations in the later stages of the disease.

How is ARMD treated.

Being a degenerative disease, ARMD has no definite treatment. But measures are available to slow down the process and make the life of the patient as comfortable as possible. Early treatment can slow down the progression of the disease and minimize the defect. The options available are:

- Certain <u>medications</u> are directly injected into the eye after anesthetizing the eye. The injections are repeated monthly.
- A combination of injections coupled with Laser therapy is available. It is called '<u>Photo Dynamic Therapy</u>' and gives significant benefit in checking the progression of the disease.
- <u>Surgery</u> with implantation of a special type of lens in the eye is available.
- It has been found that certain <u>multi-vitamin, mineral supplements</u> are of marginal benefit in retarding the progression of the disease.
- Researchers are studying the effects of <u>Gene Therapy</u> on ARMD and hopefully this may be available as an option for the treatment of the disease.

How to prevent ARMD.

Some of the simple methods of preventing the disease are as follows:

- Total avoidance of smoking.

- Regular exercise to maintain a healthy body weight.
- A nutrient rich diet is important. Fruits and vegetables in the diet provide additional benefit in preventing the disease.
- Wearing sunglasses outdoors to protect against ultraviolet rays of the sun is advisable.
- A good control of High blood pressure and elevated cholesterol levels in blood should be ensured.
- A simple test using a chart named *Amsler Grid* is available. (*See Ref 14*).This is a self-test. The patient stares at the dot in the center of the chart for a few minutes with each eye separately. If any of the lines in the grid appear wavy or if one sees blank spots on the grid, it indicates retinal disease.

MISCELLANEOUS CONDITIONS

There are many conditions that may cause problems with eyesight as a person grows older. A few of these conditions are discussed below.

FLOATERS

The normal eyeball is filled with a transparent jelly like substance called the *Vitreous*. As a person ages, this may shrink in quantity and this can lead to seeing insect-like objects floating in front of the eye. These are noticed in bright light or outdoors on a sunny day. Occasionally bright flashes of light may occur. These may look like specks of dust in one's eye which move when the eyeball is moved. They are due to tiny, solidified particles of the vitreous filling the eye. Floaters may look like threads, black spots, clouds, or small shadows. Even though they seem to be outside in front of the eye, they are really inside the eye in the vitreous.

The floaters are part of the aging process and increase with age. They are present permanently and seen in young people too, but their numbers increase with age. Often the individual with floaters in the eye gets accustomed to it that they seem to go away after a time. Initially they are annoying for the person, but later they become 'invisible' to the person's sight as he becomes accustomed to them.

Even though floaters are benign and not of any consequence, occasionally large amounts of floaters or frequent flashes of light in the eye may indicate a more serious condition like *Retinal Detachment* or Detachment of the vitreous from the retina.

To detect eye floaters, one should look at a white paper or stare at a blank white page in one's computer screen.

Causes for Floaters: Floaters are common after the age of 50. However, patients who had cataract surgery, those with short-sightedness, with bleeding into the eye, and due to inflammation in the back of the eye. are more likely to have floaters. Diabetes and High blood pressure are two diseases that can increase the number of floaters.

How do we treat floaters.

Floaters are benign and often need no treatment. Over a period of time, the person gets adjusted to them and learns to ignore them.

Occasionally when they are too troublesome, surgery is done to remove the vitreous and fill the eyeball with a similar liquid. This being a high risk surgery is not done routinely but in selected patients only.

When should a doctor be consulted for floaters.

If the number of floaters in the eye increases suddenly, one should see the eye surgeon. Flashes of light occurring in the eye along with the floaters, presence of grey areas in front of the eye or blind spots along the field of vision need to be seen by the Ophthalmologist urgently. These can be caused by a tear in the retina or due to detachment of the retina and is an ophthalmological emergency.

<u>DRY EYES</u>

Tears are normally necessary to keep the front of the eye, which is exposed to the atmosphere, wet, and lubricated. Tears contain water, electrolytes and about 1500 types of proteins. Tears are essential to wash away any irritants that may enter the eye like dust, irritant gases, or foreign particles. Tears are also produced when one gets emotional.

As a person grows old, the quantity and quality of the tears produced is reduced. This can lead to dry eyes in elderly people seen more commonly after the age of 50.

What are the symptoms of dry eyes.

- A stinging or burning feeling in the eye especially while working with computers or watching TV.
- A gritty feeling may occur in the eye. The eye may be red in some individuals.
- The person paradoxically may develop watery eyes due to irritation of the dry eyes.
- Dry eyes makes driving difficult at night.
- Dryness of the eyes occurs when the elderly are in an air conditioned environment, or when they are exposed to wind as when traveling in an open car or motorbike. Exposure to smoke can lead to dry eyes.

Causes : Dry eyes may be caused by diseases like rheumatoid arthritis, allergies, Vitamin A deficiency and thyroid disorders. Certain medications like those used for allergies, high blood pressure, depression or Parkinson's disease may cause dry eyes. Wearing contact lenses can be a cause of dry eyes in some individuals.

What complications can occur with dry eyes

- As tears give a protective coating on the surface of the eye, lack of tears can lead to eye infections.

- Dry eyes can lead to damage to the cornea of the eye and occasionally lead to corneal ulcers.
- As the person with dry eyes finds it extremely difficult to perform normal tasks like reading and sewing, the quality of life can be affected in them.

Treatment & Prevention: Over the counter eye drops – *Artificial Tears* – are available and may be instilled into the eye four to five times a day to reduce the irritation and dryness. The cause for the dryness, if detected, should be addressed. Similarly, any disease causing dryness of eyes should be properly treated. Wearing goggles while traveling in an open car is advisable.

There are medications which can increase tear production and nasal sprays are available to increase tears. Other methods used by the Ophthalmologist may be to block the ducts in the eye that drain away the tears normally, thereby making more tears to be retained in the eye. Plastic surgery may be needed in some patients if there is abnormality of the eyelids causing the eyes to dry up.

Mild massage of the eyes and warm compresses are of use in treating dry eyes. Washing the eyes with water many times a day is helpful.

Omega 3 fatty acids available in fish oils are helpful in keeping the eyes lubricated. Using a humidifier in the room especially in winter prevents dry eyes.

Drinking enough water - 8 to 10 glasses a day, wearing wrap-around glasses, avoiding exposure to wind and smoke, getting enough sleep of 6- 8 hours a day, avoiding continuous use of computer without breaks, or watching TV for long periods are needed to prevent dry eyes.

DIABETIC RETINOPATHY

Diabetic retinopathy (**DR**) is seen to affect approximately one-third of those with diabetes. The American Academy of Ophthalmology puts the global burden of Diabetes mellitus at 387 million which is expected to rise to 592 million by 2035. The number of patients affected with DR globally is approximately 93 million. In the adult type of diabetes (Type 2 Diabetes) the prevalence of DR is 25.1%.

When blood sugar levels are consistently high, this can damage the delicate vessels of the *retina* of the eye. Both the eyes are involved, but one may be more affected than the other. This can lead to progressive deterioration of vision and ultimately can cause blindness.

The chances of developing DR increases with age and the duration of diabetes. Associated conditions like kidney disease, high cholesterol levels in blood and high blood sugar increase the chances of developing DR. The chronic increase in blood sugar leads to weakening of the capillaries in the retina. These capillaries rupture causing bleeding into the retina. Fluid containing proteins also may leak into the retina causing white patches in the retina which look like cotton wool. These can be seen by the eye surgeon looking into the eye. DR may cause swelling of the retina. In addition, new blood vessels grow in the retina.

What are the symptoms of DR.

Deterioration of vision is the main symptoms of DR. It may present in various ways.

- Vision becomes blurred and foggy.
- More floaters may be seen in the eye.
- Poor night vision occurs and leads to difficulty in driving and performing tasks in dim light.
- Colors may appear faded. Objects may not be clear.
- Blank or dark areas may be seen in the field of vision.
- The symptoms often affect both eyes but may be more in one eye compared to the other.

How is Diabetic retinopathy diagnosed.
There are many tests to detect DR.

The Ophthalmologist uses eye drops to dilate the *pupil* of the eye and looks into the eye using an instrument called the Ophthalmoscope. The blood vessels in the retina, the bleeding into the retina and the white patches are clearly seen on ophthalmoscopy.

The retina can be scanned using an instrument and this Retinal Scan gives more details about the retina to the eye surgeon.

A bright yellow dye called fluorescein is injected into a vein in the arm. This dye is seen in the small blood vessels in the retina and can be photographed to get a clear picture of the blood vessels and bleeding in the retina.

How is DR treated.

The most important aspect of treating DR is keeping the blood sugar and blood pressure of the patient under control. In early stages of the disease, no active treatment is needed.

In later stages of the disease, injections maybe given into the eye which prevent the growth of new blood vessels and thereby prevent complications like bleeding into the retina.

Another treatment available is the Laser treatment where the leaking of blood and fluid into the retina from the abnormal vessels are treated with laser. It is also called *Photocoagulation* treatment. Laser treatment is used to shrink the abnormally growing blood vessels in the retina.

When there is bleeding into the vitreous, it can be removed by surgery along with any scar tissue present in the retina.

How can DR be prevented.

The main method of preventing diabetic retinopathy is keeping the patient's blood sugar, blood pressure and blood cholesterol within normal levels by proper treatment. To this end the following measures must be adopted.

- Eating a healthy 'Diabetic diet' is most important. A dietician's help may be sought for this.
- Adequate and regular exercise at least 150 minutes daily is

advised. Simple exercises like walking, swimming, cycling etc., are advised. When DR is diagnosed, strength bearing and heavy resistance exercises like weight lifting should be avoided as this can cause bleeding into the eye.

- <u>Smoking</u> must be totally given up and <u>alcohol</u> intake should be moderated.
- <u>Regular check up with the Ophthalmologist</u> is needed to observe the progression of the disease. An annual retinal screening of the eye is mandatory in any patient with long standing diabetes. Any abrupt changes noticed in vision should at once be brought to the notice of the Ophthalmologist.

<u>RETINAL DETACHMENT</u>

The normal retina is attached to the back of the eyeball all along its inner border. When it separates from its attachment to the eyeball, it is called ***Retinal Detachment*** (**RD**). It can occur in old age and also in the young. It is a serious condition and if not treated in time can lead to severe impairment of vision or blindness.

One type of RD is when there is a tear in the retina and the gel like vitreous filling the eyeball leaks out between the retina and the eyeball causing it to separate from its attachment to the back of the eyeball. This is the common type seen in the elderly individuals.

Another type of RD is when scar tissue formed in the retina as in Diabetic Retinopathy pulls the retina away from its anchorage to the eyeball and causes it to separate from its attachment to the eyeball.

The third type of RD is when the retina detaches because fluid collects behind the retina and pushes it forward, without any tear in it. This can occur in eye injuries when blood can collect behind the retina and raise it from its attachment. It may occur in certain inflammations and in tumors of the eye. RD can occur as a part of Age Related Macular Degeneration.

What are the Risk Factors for developing RD.

There are many factors which place a person at risk for developing RD.

- Short-sightedness or *Myopia* is an important cause that can lead to RD later in life. 67% of people who have RD are myopic.
- Injury to the eye can lead to RD.
- Those with family members who had RD.
- Diabetes is a risk factor in the development of RD.
- Surgery for cataract, glaucoma and other eye disorders can rarely cause RD as a complication.
- RD in one eye can lead to RD in the other eye too.

What are the symptoms of RD.

There are a few symptoms which indicate the presence of RD.

- In the early stages of mild RD, there may be no symptoms.
- Seeing flashes of light ("seeing stars") after an injury to the eye may be a symptom of RD. The flashes are better seen when the eyes are closed and are seen towards the sides of the eye. Seeing floaters in the eye may be a symptom of RD.
- In some patients, it may appear as a permanent dark shadow on one side or the periphery of the eye.
- Retinal detachment is usually painless and hence the patient may not seek immediate help for the condition.

Retinal detachment is diagnosed by the Ophthalmologist in the same way as in Diabetic retinopathy. Ophthalmoscopy and scanning of the retina are employed to diagnose the condition.

The Treatment of RD is mainly surgical or with Laser therapy. The Ophthalmologist will decide on the optimal type of treatment needed for the patient and advise accordingly. The surgery is a delicate one and post operative care is extremely important. Air travel and traveling to high altitudes may have to be avoided after the surgery. Vigorous exercises should be avoided.

Prevention of Retinal Detachment is important in certain special medical conditions like Diabetes and Short-sightedness (Myopia). These patients must have eye examinations at regular intervals by their eye surgeon.

Diabetics should always strive to keep their blood sugar will under control. Protection of the eye should be ensured with goggles whenever any risky activities are being done (Carpentry, Welding etc.) or during certain sports. Vigorous and strenuous exercises should be avoided in diabetics to prevent retinopathy.

Any symptoms like floaters or flashes of light should be promptly brought to the notice of the Ophthalmologist.

GENERAL PRECAUTIONS FOR EYE HEALTH

Seniors with poor vision should take certain precautions. The deterioration of vision in the elderly may often go unrecognized by other family members and may not be reported by the person. Some of the indicators of failing vision are:

- Frequent falls may indicate that they are not able to see the floor or steps properly.
- Bumping into things while moving around the home may indicate impaired vision.
- Inability to tolerate bright light and glare is also a symptom of visual impairment in the elderly.
- While reading or doing close work, they may tend to squint or bend their heads to focus on the nearby objects.
- Some elders may totally give up activities like sewing, reading, or writing as it becomes a tedious and stressful task for them.
- When they try to reach for an object, they may not be able to do so as they cannot focus their eyes properly on the article. This may be noticed by the relative or caregiver.

Make your life easier when you are old.

A gradual deterioration of vision may occur and often the elderly may not even be aware that they are entering this phase in life. Some preventive and precautionary measures are well worth adopting in these circumstances.

1. **Ensure Good Lighting.** A well-lit glare free lighting should be ensured for the elderly. Indoor lights should be kept switched on during daytime especially if the interior of the home is dark as in winter and rainy days. A table lamp may

be supplemented for reading or working at the table or for close work like knitting, sewing etc. For those bibliophiles who cannot read, audiobooks are available now a days.

2. **Ensure safety to prevent falls**. Poor lighting is one of the reasons for falls in elderly individuals. (See section on *Falls in the Elderly- Book 1*). To prevent this, night lamps must be provided in the bedrooms, hallways, and toilets of the elderly. Other precautions to prevent falls should be taken. Corridors should be well-lit.

3. **Contrasting colors**. To ensure easy vision, contrasting colors should be used for towels, rugs, carpets etc. White towels may be used in the bathroom against a dark wall. Light colored rugs and carpets may be used when the flooring is dark colored. The edges of steps may be highlighted with a contrasting color for the visually impaired elderly to identify them easily.

4. **Re-organization of items at home**. Large stickers and labels may be used for items of medical use and in the kitchen for ease of identification. The writings should be large, preferably in capital letters using a dark colored (black) marker pen. Other items like keys, mobile phone, wallet, jewelry etc., may be placed in baskets or trays and placed on the table, dresser, or bedside of the individual. A wider bed may be provided to prevent accidental falls at night. A lower cot may be used. Their room should not be cluttered with furniture, to avoid stumbling at night. The sharp edges of furniture or A/C unit may be padded to prevent accidental injury.

5. **Magnification**. Magnification will be needed for patients with low vision. To this end, devices which provide magnification may be used. Reading material should be of large print. These are available in libraries and in bookshops. eBooks are ideal as the magnification and contrast can be

increased as desired. Special cheque books, calendars, watches, clocks etc., are available for people with visual impairment. Spectacle mounted magnifiers are now available which can help them perform close up tasks. Hand held magnifiers for reading price tags, instructions in medicine bottles etc., are available. *I received a useful tip from an elderly gentleman who had devised his own method of magnification. While shopping, he takes a photo of the price tag or medicine instruction in his smart phone and enlarges it on his screen to read it with ease. A real innovation!*

6. **Moral Support**. Providing moral support to the elderly individual with visual impairment is very important. They often tend to become lonely and depressed as their world gets limited and activities restricted. The elderly individual should be included in the conversation at home and be encouraged to eat with others at the table. They should not be given the impression that they have been sidelined. The elderly should be encouraged to talk to other family members and friends who visit them.

7. **Other General Tips**. More pointers for elders to avoid visual problems are given below.

- Use sunglasses with ultraviolet filters. Wraparound sunglasses are ideal.
- A wide brimmed hat becomes handy while outdoors in the sun as it avoids direct sunlight into the eyes.
- A good nutritious diet is essential. Fruits and vegetables must be part of the diet. Colorful fruits and vegetables provide vitamins and essential antioxidants like Lutein and Zeaxanthin which are said to lower the risk of eye problems in old age.
- Enough sleep should be ensured as one gets old. Six to eight hours of sleep is ideal.

- While working closely or reading, frequent breaks should be taken. While working with the computer one should take frequent breaks to look out through the window or focus on an object far away from the screen for a few minutes before resuming work.
- The work space of the elderly person should be brightly and adequately lit.
- Elderly persons should get a yearly eye checkup and not ignore any of the warning signs that may indicate an impending visual disaster.

Driving safety in the elderly.

Many elderly people live alone and have to drive to get their provisions other chores done. Some may still be working if their vision is only mildly impaired. Day time vision may not be impaired to a great extent, but night vision may be seriously impaired. In these circumstances, it is essential to take some precautions. In some individuals, the driving ability is affected early even though significant symptoms of impaired vision may be lacking.

They may not be able to see the road signs properly and clearly. The instrument panel in the car may not be clearly visible to them. They may have poor night vision due to various eye conditions. In some elders, side vision or peripheral vision is poor and they may not be able to perceive a car or objects at the sides. They find it difficult to judge distances and speed of the vehicle. There may occasionally be changes in recognizing colors which can lead to misinterpretation of traffic signals and signs.

What should the elderly do to drive safely.

- The elderly should drive safely and at slow speeds. It is better to avoid highways and freeways whenever possible.
- They should endeavor to limit their driving to day time only. Night driving should be avoided as far as possible.

- At intersections, the person should be very cautious and check all sides before crossing the intersection.
- They should avoid wearing sunglasses if vision is poor and avoid glasses which are covered at the sides.
- If there are driving courses for senior citizens available in their city, they should enroll and learn safe driving for elders.
- An annual eye examination should be done for the elderly who continue to drive to rule out any new developments in their vision. The advice of the Ophthalmologist should be sought for continued driving.

Resources

1 What is Presbyopia – Boyd. K. 2022 *American Academy of Ophthalmology* .
https://www.aao.org/eye-health/diseases/what-is-presbyopia

2. Aging and your eyes – *National Institute on Aging 2022*
https://www.nia.nih.gov/health/aging-and-your-eyes

3. Presbyopia – *Mayo Clinic 2021.*
https://www.mayoclinic.org/diseases-conditions/presbyopia/symptoms-causes/syc-20363328

4. Presbyopia – *Cleveland Clinic 2020.*
https://my.clevelandclinic.org/health/diseases/8577-presbyopia

5. **20** foods that are rich in vitamin A – *Healthline 2022.*
https://www.healthline.com/nutrition/foods-high-in-vitamin-a

6.Eye problems : What to expect as you age.
https://www.webmd.com/eye-health/vision-problems-aging-adults

7 .Cataract, Causes, Symptoms and Treatment. Neely DE. 2022 *Orbis International.*
https://www.orbis.org/en/avoidable-blindness/cataracts?gclid=CjwKCAjw2OiaBhBSEiwAh2ZSP-hrLwhVgbWKL_mvQlUxrycPEbTLtV8eiB_VkvJM60HJOVeAzePp3BoCVVcQAvD

8. Cataracts – *National Eye Institute*
https://www.nei.nih.gov/learn-about-eye-health/eye-conditions-and-diseases/cataracts

9. How can I prevent cataracts – WebMD - Whitney Seltman OD
https://www.webmd.com/eye-health/cataracts/how-can-i-prevent-cataracts

10. What are the symptoms of glaucoma Fazio. D. 2022. *Glaucoma Research Foundation.*

https://glaucoma.org/what-are-the-symptoms-of-glaucoma/

11. Glaucoma, Causes, Symptoms and Treatment – Neely DE. 2022. *Orbis International*

https://www.orbis.org/en/avoidable-blindness/
glaucoma?gclid=EAIaIQobChMI9ZCEj96C-
wIViRXUAR0Bcw58EAAYAyAAEgKxBvD_BwE

12. Age Related Macular Degeneration Epidemiology and Clinical Aspects Keenan TDL et al. *Adv Exp Med Biology* 2021;1256:1-31

https://pubmed.ncbi.nlm.nih.gov/33847996/

13. Age Related Macular Degeneration (AMD) *National Eye Institute* 2021

https://www.nei.nih.gov/learn-about-eye-health/eye-conditions-and-diseases/
age-related-macular-degeneration

14. Have AMD? Save your sight with an Amsler Grid. Boyd K. 2020 *American Academy of Ophthalmology*.

https://www.aao.org/eye-health/tips-prevention/facts-about-amsler-grid-daily-
vision-test

15. Eye Floaters and Flashes – Cleveland Clinic 2022.

https://my.clevelandclinic.org/health/articles/14209-floaters—flashers[1]

16. Dry Eye – *National Eye Institute* 2022.

https://www.nei.nih.gov/learn-about-eye-health/eye-conditions-and-diseases/
dry-eye

17. Diabetic Retinopathy : Fong DS et al.: *Diabetes Care* 2004;27(10):2540–2553.

https://diabetesjournals.org/care/article/27/10/2540/23256/
Diabetic-Retinopathy

18. Retinal Detachment - *National Eye Institute* – 2022.

https://www.nei.nih.gov/learn-about-eye-health/eye-conditions-and-diseases/
retinal-detachment

19. Retinal Detachment . Chang HJ et al. *Journal of the American Medical Association*. 2012;307(13):1447

https://jamanetwork.com/journals/jama/fullarticle/1148332

---

1.   https://my.clevelandclinic.org/health/articles/14209-floaters--flashers

4. DISORDERS OF THE BLOOD

Blood is a liquid tissue in the human body. It is one of the largest tissues in volume. The total volume of blood in the adult human body is about 5 liters (12 pints).

The functions of blood are as follows:

- Carries oxygen from lungs to tissues and carbon dioxide back from the tissues to the lungs.
- Transports nutrients absorbed from the digestive system to all parts of the body.
- Carries the hormones produced by the Endocrine glands to the various parts of the body where they act.
- Blood transports the cells and antibodies needed to fight infections.
- Waste products produced during metabolism of tissues are carried to the kidneys and liver to be eliminated.
- Blood plays an active role in regulating the body temperature of the individual.
- Regulating the fluid and electrolyte balance in the body is an important function of blood.
- Loss of blood when the blood vessels are breached is prevented by forming a blood clot which seals the defect in the vessel, thus preventing blood loss from the body.

Blood is composed of four main components – the liquid part called *Plasma*, the **Red Blood Cells,** the **White Blood Cells**, and the **Platelets**. The plasma comprises 55% of the blood whereas the cells form the rests 45%.

Blood is formed in the bone marrow which occupies the hollow inner portion of long bones, vertebrae, ribs, pelvis, and skull. The marrow is the spongy tissue that fills these marrow spaces in the bones. The blood cells are derived from a primitive cell called the *Stem Cell* which can differentiate into all types of blood cells.

<u>**Blood Components - Composition**</u>

Plasma. This is the liquid content of the blood, 90% of which is water. The rest of plasma is formed of Proteins, Fats, Sugar, *Electrolytes*, and minerals dissolved in it. The blood cells are suspended in the plasma.

Red Blood Cells (RBC). The RBC is red in color. It has the shape of a Biconcave Disc or looks like a doughnut – disc shaped with a central indentation. Looking at it from the side, an RBC would look like a dumbbell. The red color is due to the presence of a red iron containing pigment called **_Hemoglobin_**. The hemoglobin is the component of the RBC that carries oxygen and carbon dioxide to and fro between the lungs and tissues of the body.

The RBCs are produced in the bone marrow from the stem cells and mature within 7 days and are released into the blood stream. They remain in the blood stream for about 120 days. The RBCs form a major part of the cells in blood constituting 40-45% of the volume of blood and this gives blood its red color.

The normal RBC count in men is 4.0 to 5.9 million cells per microliter of blood and in women is 3.8 to 5.2 million cells per microliter.

White Blood Cells. (WBC). The WBCs form only about 1% of the volume of blood but are a very important component of blood as they are the warriors protecting the body against any infection by _microorganisms_. They are of different types and each has a specific function protecting the body against external "invaders" like bacteria, viruses, and _allergens_.

Of the WBCs, the **_Neutrophils_** are the ones which form the majority. They are the cells which immediately reach any site of infection to devour the bacteria or viruses. They have a very short lifespan of one day. (**Figure 4**).

Another type of WBCs named **_Lymphocytes_** and are involved in producing antibodies which attack and destroy bacteria, viruses, and other foreign materials.

There are other types of WBCs which form a very minor percentage of the WBCs. **Basophils** are cells which attack allergens and parasites which infest the body. **Eosinophils** are white cells which are also involved against allergens and parasites. **Plasma cells** are another type of white cells. They are produced in bone marrow but are not found normally in peripheral blood. They are found in the bone marrow and lymphatic tissues. They secrete antibodies or _immunoglobulins_.

The normal WBC count is 4500 to 11,000 cells per microliter.

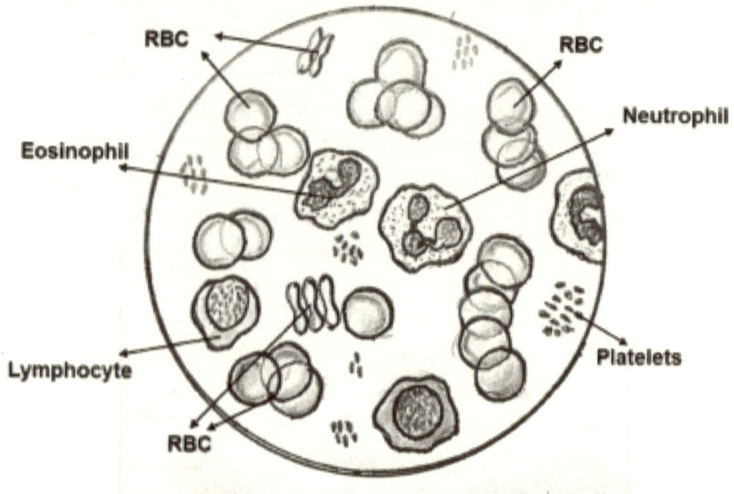

Figure 4

Platelets. They are much smaller than the WBCs or RBCs. These are very tiny, colorless cells, which are small pieces broken off from a larger cell. These are the main cells concerned with blood clotting. Platelets accumulate at the site of injury of a blood vessel, stick together and form clumps on which the blood clot develops. Thus, they are a defense mechanism to prevent blood loss. The normal platelet count in blood is <u>150,000 to 450,000 per microliter.</u>

Lymphatic System

The lymphatic system consists of a network of vessels, lymph nodes, and ducts which ultimately join the circulatory system and empty their contents into blood. This system of vessels which is rampant in all tissues helps to maintain the fluid balance in the body. The spleen is an important organ of the lymphatic system.

Excess fluid from the tissues and small particulate matter entering the body are collected by these vessels. The fluid in the lymphatic vessels is called *Lymph*. The lymphatic system also helps the body's defense mechanism by producing white blood cells (Lymphocytes and Plasma cells) which manufacture antibodies and thus help fight infection. Thus, the lymphatic system is a 'drainage system' which carries its contents into blood.

The lymphatic system also helps in the absorption of digested fat from the intestines. The fatty acids which are produced when fat is digested are carried by the lymphatic vessels to be ultimately emptied into blood.

When blood circulates and reaches the tissues, the plasma along with the nutrients, oxygen, minerals, etc., seeps into the tissues to supply them. The fluid which thus seeps out is removed by the lymphatic system of vessels and ultimately drained back into the blood, thus keeping the fluid balance in the tissues normal. The smaller lymphatic vessels join to form larger vessels which ultimately drain into the veins inside the chest.

Many organs of the body have these lymphatic tissues. The Thymus, which is an organ, situated in the chest behind the breastbone (sternum) is one such organ.

Lymphatic tissues are also present in the numerous Lymph nodes (about 500-600) which are situated in many parts of the body along the path of the lymphatic vessels. On the surface of the body, the lymph nodes can be seen or felt in the neck, above the collar bone, in the armpits, knees and the groins. They are also present deep in the chest and abdomen. The lymphatic tissues are present in the spleen, tonsils, in the small intestines and the appendix in the large intestine. The lymphatic vessels carry the infectious agents or foreign material which may enter the body. These are trapped in the lymph nodes and destroyed. That is why the lymph nodes become swollen when there is an infection.

The spleen in a lymphatic organ found in the left upper part of the abdomen behind the stomach under the rib cage. The spleen is supplied by an artery which brings blood in and a vein which takes out the blood. The spleen functions as a filter for the blood and removes any bacteria which may be present in blood and the old blood cells. The spleen also produces lymphocytes and plasma cells and thus actively participates in the defense mechanism of the body.

Blood is a tissue composed of 55% liquid called Plasma and 45% of cells. An adult body contains about 5 liters of blood. As a person ages, the chances of developing diseases of the blood increase.

The elderly are disadvantaged by the fact that they are frail, poorly tolerate treatment like chemotherapy for cancers, develop more side effects with medications and have low chances of success with treatment.

The blood diseases common in old age are Anemia and Blood Cancer. There are other disorders like low platelets (*Thrombocytopenia*) which are uncommon. As one ages, the infection fighting capacity of WBCs decreases. The blood clotting factors which are needed for normal clotting of blood *increase* as one ages and this may result in abnormal clotting of blood in parts of the body.

ANEMIA

Anemia is the commonest disease of blood in the elderly. The term 'Anemia' indicates a reduction in Red blood cells (RBC) or a deficiency of Hemoglobin in blood. *The World Health Organization has defined anemia as a value of hemoglobin below **13 grams/100 ml in men or 12 grams/100 ml in women.***

The space in the bone marrow occupied by blood producing cells decreases as one grows older. While 90% of the marrow space is filled with blood producing cells in the newborn, it decreases to 50% at the age of 30 and to 30% at the age of 70.

What causes Anemia in the Elderly.

There are many causes for the development of anemia in the elderly. Some of the common causes are as follows.

- <u>Chronic diseases and infections</u> can lead to anemia. Chronic Kidney disease commonly causes anemia. Hypothyroidism, and hyperthyroidism are associated with anemia. Thyroid disease is a common cause of anemia in the elderly and constitutes almost 30-45% of cases.
- <u>Iron Deficiency</u> causes anemia in the elderly. Iron is a component of Hemoglobin and is an essential element in blood formation. Iron deficiency is the second commonest cause and is seen in about 15-30% of those with anemia. This can occur due to chronic blood loss as occurs with frequent intake of pain relieving medications like aspirin or NSAIDs, inadequate intake, or poor absorption of iron from the gut.
- <u>Vitamin B12</u> is another nutrient whose deficiency can lead to anemia. Inadequate intake of the vitamin may occur in vegetarians and vegans. Surgery on the stomach and intestines can lead to poor absorption of the vitamin.
- <u>Folic Acid</u> is a vitamin whose deficiency can lead to anemia.

- <u>Blood loss</u> occurring from bleeding from the gastrointestinal tract is an important cause which may go unrecognized. Peptic ulcers, polyps, piles, and cancers in the GI tract may bleed and lead to anemia.
- <u>Other minerals</u> like zinc, magnesium, selenium, and copper are also needed for blood formation and may cause anemia when deficient.

What are the symptoms of anemia.

There are many nonspecific symptoms which may occur when a patient is anemic.

- Fatigue and tiredness. Lack of energy and poor concentration are common.
- Shortness of breath may occur as the person's blood has a lower capacity to transport oxygen to the tissues. Hence the patient feels breathless even with minor exertion.
- Occasionally they feel palpitations, as the heart overworks to circulate blood to the tissues.
- Dizziness and giddiness may be felt. The patient may feel a pulsating sensation in the ear.
- Fainting attacks may occur is some patients if the anemia is severe.
- The patient has a pale and sallow complexion. The tongue and the inside of the lower eyelid are pale compared to their normal pink color.
- Difficulty in swallowing and hair loss may occur in some patients.
- Anemic persons may have a strange habit called '**Pica**'. It is the desire to eat unusual things like raw rice, paper, chalk, or soil.
- If there is bleeding in the GI tract, the stools may have a black color like tar due to altered blood.
- Swelling of the legs may occur in certain cases of severe

anemia.

- The abdomen may be swollen in some if there is enlargement of the liver and spleen.

How can anemia affect a person's life.

Anemia may bring about many changes in the life of the individual.

- Anemia decreases the quality of life of the person and makes him frailer.
- As the anemia increases, the person feels giddy and unsteady leading to falls and fractures in the elderly.
- Anemia may aggravate previously existing diseases, especially heart diseases.
- Dementia, depression, and sleeplessness may accompany anemia in the elderly.
- Anemia often increases the hospital stay after surgery or after an infection.

Diagnosis.

The physician makes a diagnosis of anemia by examining the patient's clinical features like the presence of pallor, enlarged liver or spleen and other clinical features.

Blood tests are important in diagnosis. A blood smear taken from a finger prick examined under the microscope in a laboratory gives a quick diagnosis. A test named '**Complete Blood Count**' (CBC) is done where the number of RBCs, WBCs, platelets, Hemoglobin concentration, and many other important parameters are measured in blood. This gives a comprehensive understanding regarding the status of the blood.

Others detailed tests may be needed in blood to determine the levels of various factors like iron and vitamins. Tests of liver and kidney function are also done.

A bone marrow biopsy is done by taking a small bit of tissue from the bone marrow and subjecting it to laboratory tests to determine the cause and type of anemia. **How is anemia treated.**

The mainstay of treatment is determining the cause of anemia and treating it. Iron, Vitamin, or mineral deficiencies are treated by replacing the appropriate item orally through tablets, syrups or by injections.

If bleeding from the GI tract is the cause of blood loss, the cause is identified and treated appropriately.

A good nutritious diet should be ensured containing vegetables, fruits, and nuts. Lean meat and fish are suggested to increase the production of blood. Vegetarians are encouraged to eat more of grains, cereals, and tofu.

In severe anemia blood transfusion is given where the RBCs isolated from donated blood are transfused into the patient.

In chronic kidney disease, a hormone named *Erythropoietin* is given as injections as this stimulates the bone marrow to produce more RBCs.

A regular supplement of Vitamins and Minerals are advised by the physician in the elderly to prevent anemia and other nutritional disorders.

How can Anemia in the Elderly be prevented.

A healthy diet as mentioned earlier is the most important aspect of preventing anemia. A diet which includes dark green leafy vegetables like spinach and kale, lean meat, liver, poultry, lentils, beans, soya, tofu, dark chocolate, dry fruits, and quinoa is a rich source of iron.

Some of the cereals and flour available in the market are fortified with iron or folic acid and provide adequate intake of these nutrients.

It is safer to avoid contact with heavy metals like lead which can cause anemia. Human contact with lead occurs while using lead containing paints, pipes, pottery, battery recycling etc. It is also found in some medicines used in Alternative medicine. Lead mining and smelting facilities may cause exposure to lead. Lead can contaminate water also.

Other measures in the prevention of anemia are good dental hygiene to help proper food intake, adequate water intake and maintaining a healthy lifestyle free of alcohol and smoking.

BLOOD CANCER

The term 'Blood Cancer' indicates an unusual and abnormal proliferation of the cells in the bone marrow and/or the lymphoid tissue leading to an increase in the number of abnormal cells in the blood. This occurs because of abnormal changes in the *DNA* of the blood cells. Such a change in the DNA is called *Mutation* and leads to an abnormal colony of cells which multiply without any control, giving rise to the cancer.

This abnormal proliferation is seen in the white blood cells and can be of three types.

Leukemia which is due to an abnormal proliferation of the WBCs in the bone marrow. These abnormal WBCs cannot function normally to fight infection and hence are not functionally useful. The abnormal multiplication of these cells in the marrow crowds out the normal RBCs and platelets which may decrease in number causing anemia and decrease in platelets.

Lymphoma is a type of blood cancer that starts in the lymphatic system of the body. The normal cells produced here are the lymphocytes. In lymphoma, the cells are abnormal and hence they are not able to fight infection and do not produce effective antibodies.

Multiple Myeloma is a type of blood cancer where plasma cells increase in number. The cells are abnormal and hence cannot produce effective antibodies to fight infection.

LEUKEMIA

Leukemia indicates a cancer of the white blood cells. There are mainly two types of leukemia – **Myeloid Leukemia** and **Lymphocytic Leukemia.** These can be **Acute** when the onset is rapid and often leading to a fatal end, or **Chronic** where the course of disease is long drawn.

ACUTE MYELOID LEUKEMIA. (AML)

It affects a group of white cells in the marrow known as myeloid cells. These are mainly the Neutrophils. It is also called **Acute Myelogenous Leukemia**. It has a rather abrupt onset and a rapid progression.

AML often presents with symptoms of fever, tiredness, breathlessness, *pallor,* repeated infections especially of the lung, easy bruising of the skin and bleeding from the gums or nose. Men are affected more. Previous exposure to radiation, benzene chemicals, smoking or chemotherapy for other cancers can increase the risk of developing AML. The risk of this cancer is high in certain genetic diseases like *Downs Syndrome.*

The disease is diagnosed by examining the blood and the bone marrow biopsy in the lab.

The mainstay of treatment is chemotherapy to kill the cancer cells. The aim of treatment is to first control the acute symptoms and induce a *remission.* Following this medications are given for maintenance of the remission.

Bone marrow transplantation is a mode of treatment for all leukemias and is used in AML.

ACUTE LYMPHOCYTIC LEUKEMIA (ALL)

This is the type of leukemia where the white cells called Lymphocytes multiply to produce large numbers of abnormal cells which are functionally inactive. Hence they are not able to perform their designated function of producing antibodies and fighting infections.

ALL is more common in children but may occur in adults and elderly where the treatment is more difficult. The symptoms are almost similar to that of AML, but in addition, lymph nodes may be enlarged in the groin, armpit, neck, and inside the chest and abdomen.

The disease is diagnosed by examining a sample of blood and a biopsy specimen from the bone marrow.

In children the disease is more amenable to treatment but in adults and the elderly, treatment may not be very effective. As in AML, initially a remission is achieved with chemotherapy followed by maintenance therapy.

Chemotherapy, Targeted therapy, Immunotherapy, Radiation therapy and bone marrow transplantation are the treatments available. In older adults, the treatment may not yield satisfactory results as in children and often the complications of treatment are higher.

CHRONIC MYELOID LEUKEMIA (CML)

This is a disease of older adults. It is rare in children. CML is not a common leukemia. The white cells in the marrow multiply without control. The abnormal cells spill over into the blood. The onset of the disease is slow and it progresses very slowly and may not be detected in early stages as symptoms are minimal or absent.

Initially the disease may only cause tiredness, anemia, and breathlessness. Often the disease may be detected on routine examination of blood.

Treatment is by chemotherapy and occasionally by bone marrow transplantation.

CHRONIC LYMPHOCYTIC LEUKEMIA (CLL)

In this type of leukemia, abnormal lymphocytes multiply in large numbers. This is often seen in elderly individuals and has a slowly advancing course.

Weight loss, tiredness, breathlessness, painless enlargement of the lymph nodes in the armpit, groin, neck, and other areas of the body are seen. The abdomen may appear swollen if the spleen is enlarged. A low grade fever with sweating at night may be present in some. As their immunity is low, they may have frequent infections especially of the lung.

CLL is diagnosed by examining the peripheral blood. A smear from the blood is tested in the laboratory and this shows large numbers of abnormal lymphocytes. A bone marrow biopsy supplements the diagnosis. The enlarged lymph node can be removed and examined microscopically to see the proliferation of abnormal cells. Other tests to determine the type of cell may be done to plan appropriate treatment.

In early stages of the disease, the doctor may opt not to start any treatment but keep the patient under constant observation. Later on, if the disease increases in severity, treatment is instituted in the form of Chemotherapy, targeted therapy, immunotherapy, or bone marrow transplantation depending on the severity of the disease and the general physical condition of the patient.

MULTIPLE MYELOMA (MM)

This is a blood cancer of the elderly occurring at an average age of 70. This cancer is due to the uncontrolled multiplication of an abnormal clone of plasma cells. The normal plasma cell, which is a variant of the WBC, is concerned with making antibodies (*Immunoglobulins*). It is known that a single plasma cell can secrete hundreds of molecules of antibodies in *one second*!

In Multiple Myeloma, the immunoglobulins manufactured by these plasma cells are abnormal and are called **Myeloma Proteins** (M-proteins).

In the US, 15% of blood cancers is multiple myeloma and of these roughly 1/3 of patients are above the age of 75.

What are the Clinical Features of Multiple Myeloma.

- About 30% of patients with MM do not have any symptoms in early stages of the disease. About 1/3 of the patients are diagnosed with MM only when they develop a fracture of a bone due to the disease.
- Severe tiredness, and headaches may occur. Numbness of the limbs is often a common feature.
- Repeated infections like pneumonia may occur in the elderly as their immune status is reduced. A low grade fever may be present in some.

- Bone pain is often an important symptom. It is seen in almost half of the patients with MM. It may present as back pain or pain in the spine, ribs, or long bones. The multiplication of the tumor cells in the marrow weakens the bones leading to abnormal fractures which may occur with trivial trauma.

- An unexplained loss of weight is seen in many patients.

- Some develop nausea and vomiting with loss of appetite which are due to the high calcium levels in blood. (*Hypercalcemia*).

- A decrease in blood platelets may cause easy bruising and occasionally bleeding from gums or nose.

- Almost 40% of patients with MM develop kidney failure as a complication.

- Severe anemia occurs in some patients because the bone marrow is filled with abnormal plasma cells which displace the cells producing the RBCs.

- The spinal cord inside the vertebral column may be compressed by either fracture of the vertebrae or due to clumps of abnormal tumor cells leading to weakness of the limbs and other neurological disorders.

How is Multiple Myeloma diagnosed.

The following investigations are done when MM is suspected in a patient.

The smear taken from blood may show abnormal plasma cells occasionally. They are not numerous as occurs in leukemia. But the smear may show a decrease in platelets and changes due to anemia. The RBCs are seen to be stacked together in long chains which are called "**rouleaux**" formation. It appears like a stack of doughnuts. This is due to the abnormal proteins produced by the plasma cells which circulate in blood causing the RBCs to stick to each other.

Blood tests for Kidney function may indicate kidney damage. The serum calcium is increased above normal levels (*Hypercalcemia*).

Electrophoresis of *plasma* or *serum* is used to identify the abnormal proteins produced by the plasma cells. In this test an electric current is used to separate the different proteins in plasma, as they move at different speeds in an electrical field depending on the size of their molecules. The abnormal M-protein can be identified by this procedure.

A Complete blood count shows the presence of anemia and a shortage of platelets and other WBCs.

Examination of the urine also shows the abnormal proteins in MM.

A bone marrow biopsy gives the definite diagnosis. Clumps of abnormal plasma cells are seen displacing the other blood cell producing tissues.

X-rays of the spine, skull and pelvis are usually done. These show punched out shadows in the bones as if there are 'holes' in the bones. These are due to erosion of the bones by the clumps of abnormal plasma cells.

Additional tests like MRI and PET scan are done at times to know the extent of bone involvement in the body.

How is Multiple Myeloma treated.

Even though the disease is not fully curable, remission can be obtained in most patients with the advances in management of myeloma in recent times.

- If the patient does not have many symptoms, routinely detected myeloma may not be treated in early stages.
- To obtain a remission, Chemotherapy, Targeted therapy, and Immunotherapy are given.
- Steroids and other medications are used in some patients.
- Bone marrow transplantation is done in comparatively younger patients or the elderly with good physical fitness.

Supportive Therapy.

Supportive therapy aims at relieving the symptoms and complications of the disease.

- Patients with bone pain often need pain relieving medications. Some patients are relieved with mild medications whereas others may need stronger ones like opioids or injections for the relief of pain. Occasionally, radiation is given to relieve bone pain. Bone fractures are dealt with by the Orthopedic surgeon.
- Kidney failure needs the intervention of a *Nephrologist* who plans the treatment of kidney failure. Some patients may need chronic *dialysis* to overcome the failure.
- Infections, when present are treated with antibiotics.
- Anemia is treated with blood transfusions.
- When platelets are low causing bleeding complications, transfusion of platelets is given.

Survival with Multiple Myeloma.

Multiple Myeloma is an incurable disease. The *Oncologist* often aims at remission in the acute stage of the disease. Modern methods of treatment has increased the survival after MM. Bone marrow transplantation, which is often advised for those below 65 years of age increases survival.

Survival in multiple myeloma and other cancers is often reported as a *"Five-year survival"*. This indicates the percentage of patients who survive at the end of five years. The 5-year survival depends on the stage of the disease. In very early stages there may be a 90-100% survival at the end of 5 years, whereas in severe cases the 5-year survival is only 10-15%.

LYMPHOMA.

Lymphomas are cancers which begin in the lymphatic system. The lymphatic system is a subsystem of the circulatory system. The white blood cells which produce antibodies – the Lymphocytes, are produced in the lymphatic system. The lymph nodes which are seen all along the lymphatic system are the first line of defense in the body against invading *microorganisms*. The lymphatic system exists in the spleen, thymus, bone marrow and other organs.

When the cells in the lymphatic system turn cancerous, it is called **Lymphoma**. The cells which become cancerous are the Lymphocytes. There are two types of lymphoma which are common.

1. Non-Hodgkin Lymphoma, which is seen more in the elderly, aged 60-80 years and is more common in men.
2. Hodgkin Lymphoma which is commonly seen in two age groups – those between 20-30 years and in those above 65 years.

What are the symptoms of Lymphoma.

The most important symptom is the enlargement of the lymph nodes. The person notices painless enlargement of the lymph nodes in the neck, above the collar bone, below the lower jaw, axilla, and groin.

Severe tiredness which is a feature in most of the cancers is seen in lymphoma.

Unexplained weight loss and loss of appetite are other symptoms.

A low grade fever may be seen in some patients. Night sweats are frequent in many patients.

Shortness of breath due to the associated anemia is often present.

Some patients develop a generalized itching all over the body without any obvious reason for it. This is due to chemicals called *Cytokines* released by the tumor and which irritate the nerves in the skin causing itching.

Some patients may develop skin rashes.

When the lymph nodes inside the chest are swollen, they may press on the windpipe or its branches and induce cough or breathlessness. Pain behind the breast bone may be felt.

What are the Risk factors for Lymphoma to develop.

There are some risk factors described which increase the chances of developing lymphoma. They are:

- **Age** itself is a risk factor. Lymphoma is common after the age of 65.
- **Gender** is mentioned as a risk factor as the disease is more common in males.
- **Whites** are more prone to lymphoma compared to African Americans and Asians.
- Some **chemicals** in insecticides and some herbicides can increase the risk of development of lymphoma. Benzene and petrochemicals are identified as risk factors.
- Some patients who have had **chemotherapy** for one type of cancer may develop lymphoma years later.
- **Radiation** is a risk factor. Individuals who have been exposed to radiation accidentally while working in nuclear reactor plants or those who had radiation therapy for others cancers have a higher risk of developing lymphoma later in life.
- A weak immune system as occurs in **infection with the Human Immunodeficiency Virus** (HIV or AIDS virus) can lead to lymphoma in the affected patients. Patients who have had transplanted organs are given medications to suppress their immune system to prevent rejection. These patients run the risk of developing lymphoma.
- An increased risk of lymphoma is associated with some **autoimmune diseases** like rheumatoid arthritis.
- Infection with a virus named **Epstein-Barr Virus** (EBV) which causes a disease called Infectious Mononucleosis at a younger age is a risk factor for development of lymphoma later in life.

How is Lymphoma Diagnosed.

A simple physical examination of the patient tells the doctor that lymph nodes in the body are enlarged. The doctor can feel the enlarged spleen in the abdomen. In addition, pallor, which is a feature of anemia is noticed.

A complete blood count is often done to note any abnormal cells present in blood. The test reveals anemia and reduction in the number of platelets.

Blood tests are done to assess the functions of the liver and kidneys.

A lymph node biopsy tells the doctor the details regarding the lymphoma and the type of cell in the tumor.

A chest X-ray is done to verify whether the lymph nodes in the chest are swollen or if the lungs are involved.

A bone marrow biopsy is done to assess the presence of lymphoma in the bone marrow.

Other tests like CT scan, MRI scan or PET scan may be advised by the treating doctor depending on the need.

How is Lymphoma treated.

Some lymphomas grow very slowly. In such cases, the treating doctor may not start any active treatment immediately but follow up the patient to see the further evolution of the disease.

Chemotherapy, Radiation therapy, Immunotherapy and Targeted Therapy are used in treating lymphomas.

Bone marrow transplantation is used in the treatment of lymphomas in comparatively younger and physically fit patients.

Survival in Lymphoma.

The 5- year survival depends on various factors. Those below the age of 60 have a better survival compared to those older. Those with mild disease (Stage I) affecting only a small group of lymph nodes have a better survival than those with involvement of almost all the nodes in the body (Stage IV). An overall 5-year survival rate of 70-75% is seen with most lymphomas.

THROMBOCYTOPENIA

The platelets are the smallest of the blood cells. They are really bits of cells which break off from a larger 'mother' cell in the bone marrow. The platelets are active in blood clotting which is essential to seal off any area of damage or break in a blood vessel. The platelets immediately rush to the area of damage or cut in the blood vessel, stick together and form clumps which plug the vessel to prevent bleeding. The platelets release certain substances which in turn cause clotting of blood and thus prevent further bleeding.

The platelet is also named the '*Thrombocyte*'. A decrease in platelet count in blood is called '*Thrombocytopenia*'. Hence, if the platelet count goes to very low levels, it can lead to bleeding as clotting is not effective. Thrombocytopenia is an abnormal lowering of platelet count and may be a serious and fatal disease.

In the elderly patient, thrombocytopenia may be worse owing to the presence of co-morbidities. A greater risk of bleeding due to the weakening of tissues and concomitant use of medications which may cause decrease of platelet function may create additional problems. The elderly are prone to falls and sustain injuries which increases their chances of bleeding. Poor cognitive function in the elderly may lead to poor awareness of the symptoms.

What are the causes of Thrombocytopenia.

Thrombocytopenia may be caused by many factors. Some of them are:

- Decreased production of platelets may occur in blood cancers because the cancer cells invade the bone marrow and displace the cells which give rise to the platelets.
- A decrease in platelets is seen in many viral and bacterial infections. Some of these are Dengue Fever and Hepatitis C infection.

- Chemotherapy or Radiation therapy given for other cancers may cause a decrease in the platelet count.
- Autoimmune diseases where the immune system of the body attacks the person's normal healthy cells damaging them, can affect the platelets. Platelets may decrease in diseases like Rheumatoid arthritis. Immune Thrombocytopenia (ITP) is a condition where the body attacks the healthy platelets to cause a decline in the count.
- Various medications can lead to Thrombocytopenia. Medicines like Sulfonamide drugs, Acetaminophen (*Tylenol, Panadol*), Ibuprofen (*Motrin*), Naproxen (*Naprosyn*), some antibiotics, and medications used for epilepsy can decrease platelet numbers.
- Toxic chemicals in pesticides, arsenic and benzene are known to cause thrombocytopenia.
- The presence of foreign material as in devices introduced in the blood circulation like artificial heart valves and blood vessel grafts can lead to a low platelet count.
- Heavy alcohol intake has been associated with thrombocytopenia.
- Normally, the spleen traps platelets and destroys it as the lifespan of a platelet is about ten days. An enlargement of the spleen can trap more platelets in it leading to a thrombocytopenia.

What are the symptoms of Thrombocytopenia.

The main symptom caused by a decrease in platelet count is the inability of blood to clot to prevent bleeding. Most of the symptoms are hence due to bleeding from various sites in the body.

- Spontaneous bleeding may occur into the skin giving red spots on the skin which look like insect bites. Occasionally these bleeding areas may be large especially in the arms and legs.

- An increased susceptibility to bruising is noticed even with minor trauma.
- In case of a cut or prick, the bleeding continues for prolonged periods.
- Bleeding can occur from the nose or the gums. Bleeding into the stomach leads to vomiting of blood or blood may be passed in stools.
- Bleeding from the kidneys or bladder may cause blood in the urine.
- When the bleeding occurs into the brain it presents as brain hemorrhage leading to stroke. (See Section on *Stroke in Book 1*).
- The doctor examining the patient may find these bleeding signs and find a large spleen.

How is Thrombocytopenia diagnosed.

The most important blood test is a Complete Blood Count which shows a very low Platelet Count. Often serious and fatal bleeding may occur if the counts go below 10,000 cells per microliter of blood.

A smear taken from the peripheral blood shows a very low number of platelets under the microscope. The normally seen clumps of platelets are often absent in thrombocytopenia.

A Bone marrow biopsy often confirms the presence of low platelets and identifies the cause of the thrombocytopenia.

Others tests for clotting of blood are done on a blood sample to know if the clotting of blood is impaired.

How is Thrombocytopenia treated.

- If there is a cause detected for the thrombocytopenia like a toxic chemical, medication or alcohol, the cause should be removed.
- Steroids are often helpful in immune mediated thrombocytopenia.

- A transfusion of platelets is given to the patient if the levels are low. This can be repeated till the count reaches safe levels.
- Surgery for thrombocytopenia involves surgical removal of the spleen so that the trapping and destruction of the platelets is reduced.
- The bacterial or viral infection which is the cause of the low platelet count is aggressively treated.

Precautions to be taken in an Elderly with Thrombocytopenia.

If an elderly is diagnosed with thrombocytopenia, he should take care to avoid falls and injury as the bleeding could be heavy and fatal. Any simple head injury in the elderly can lead to bleeding into the brain which is serious. If any cut or injury is causing a prolonged bleeding, pressure should be applied to the area till the bleeding stops or till medical help is sought.

Extreme caution is advised while driving and traveling and care is taken to wear the seat belt or helmet while using cars or two-wheelers. Hobbies where injuries are likely like carpentry or gardening are better avoided.

A healthy lifestyle devoid of smoking and moderation in alcohol intake are advised.

Care should be taken to preserve one's dental hygiene.

Over the counter medications, especially pain killers should be taken with caution and any medication should be taken only after consultation with one's treating physician.

Resources

1. Davidson's Principles and Practice of Medicine 23rd edition. Elsevier-2018 Chapter 23. *Hematology & Transfusion Medicine* pages 911-980.
2. Hematology in Older Persons. Ershler WB et al. *Williams Hematology* 9 Ed. Chapter 9. 2016. McGraw-Hill. https://accessmedicine.mhmedical.com/

    content.aspx?bookid=1581§ionid=94301148

3. Aging and Blood Disorders. New Perspectives. New Challenges. Bron D et al. *Hematologica* . 2015. 100 : pages 415-417.

https://www.ncbi.nlm.nih.gov/pmc/articles/PMC4380713/

1. Anemia in Elderly Persons. Olmedo K. *Medscape* 2022.

https://emedicine.medscape.com/article/1339998-overview#a1

1. Chronic Lymphocytic Leukemia. *Mayo Clinic*. 2022.

https://www.mayoclinic.org/diseases-conditions/chronic-lymphocytic-leukemia/symptoms-causes/syc-20352428

1. What to Expect with Leukemia as an Older Adult. Selchik. F *Healthline*.

https://www.healthline.com/health/leukemia/leukemia-in-elderly

1. Acute Myelogenous Leukemia. *Mayo Clinic* 2022.

https://www.mayoclinic.org/diseases-conditions/acute-myelogenous-leukemia/symptoms-causes/syc-20369109

1. About Acute Lymphocytic Leukemia. *American Cancer Society*. 2018.

https://www.cancer.org/cancer/acute-lymphocytic-leukemia/about.html

1. Multiple Myeloma in the Very Elderly Patient. Challenges and Solutions. Willan J et al. *Clin. Intervention Aging*. 2016. 11: pages 423-435.

https://www.ncbi.nlm.nih.gov/pmc/articles/PMC4839967/

1. Treatment of Multiple Myeloma in Elderly Patients. A Review of Literature and Practice Guidelines. Manapuram S, Hashmi H. *Cureus* 10(12): e3669. doi:10.7759/cureus.3669.

https://www.ncbi.nlm.nih.gov/pmc/articles/PMC6364954/

1. Lymphoma. *Centers for Disease Control & Prevention.* 2018

https://www.cdc.gov/cancer/lymphoma/index.htm

1. Platelet Disorders -Thrombocytopenia. *National, Heart, Lung & Blood Institute.* 2022.

https://www.nhlbi.nih.gov/health/thrombocytopenia

5.GYNECOLOGICAL DISORDERS

FEMALE REPRODUCTIVE SYSTEM

The main parts of the female reproductive system are the Uterus, the Ovaries, the Fallopian Tubes, and the Vagina. These constitute the female organs concerned with sexuality and reproduction. The uterus is situated in the pelvis of the female sandwiched between the urinary bladder in front and the rectum behind. The hormones secreted by the system control the menstruation in females.

The external genitals in the female are the **Vulva**. They contain two lip like vertical skin folds called the **Labia**. These protect the entry into the vagina. A thin membrane is seen at the entrance to the vagina in virgins partly covering the entrance to the vagina. It is called the **Hymen**. The urethra opens into this area in the female.

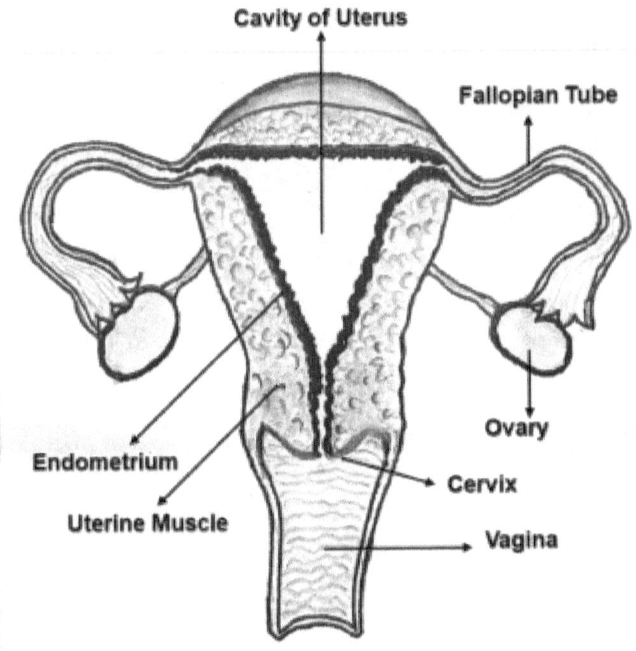

Figure 5

The external genitals or the vulva leads into the **Vagina,** which is an elastic, muscular tube which ends at the entrance of the uterus. The vagina is about 3 inches long. The vagina can dilate to accommodate the passage of the baby during delivery.

The **Cervix** is the part of the uterus which is seen at the upper end of the vagina. It has a central aperture which leads into the uterus. It is through this opening that the sperms enter the uterus during sexual intercourse. The cervix dilates during delivery to permit the baby to descend into the vagina. (**Figure 5**).

The **Uterus** or womb is the organ in the pelvis in which the baby grows. It is shaped like an inverted pear. The uterus is hollow inside and is about 3 inches long and 2 inches wide at the top. The inner lining of the uterus is called the *Endometrium*. The uterus has a thick muscle coat in its wall which can stretch to a large size during pregnancy to accommodate the growing *fetus*. The muscular coat is in the middle. This inner lining of the uterus is shed every month during menstruation and new endometrium is replaced. The endometrium is richly supplied with blood vessels.

The **Ovaries** are a pair of oval almond-shaped glands that are seen on either side of the body of the uterus. They produce the **Ova** or eggs which are released every month to be carried into the cavity of the uterus. The ovaries produce the female hormones which are released into the blood circulation.

The **Fallopian tubes** or Uterine tubes are the hollow channels through which the eggs released from the ovaries are carried to the cavity of the uterus to be fertilized by the sperms entering the uterus. They are attached to the upper part of the uterus on either side. Usually, fertilization occurs inside these tubes and the fertilized egg travels to the uterus.

Gynecological problems are common in elderly women as they would have already attained *menopause*. During the adult years, the female hormones mainly, estrogen helps to keep the vagina lubricated and well supplied with blood vessels. As aging occurs the level of estrogens produced is reduced and this leads to *atrophy* of the genitals in the woman. The external genitals hence become thinner and dry as the normal secretions dry up. The uterus shrinks in size and the inner lining of the uterus, the *Endometrium* becomes thin.

The ovaries decrease in size. The production of the two female hormones Estrogen and Progesterone by the ovaries is reduced. They also stop releasing eggs every month. Menstrual bleeding stops after menopause. Sexual intercourse becomes painful after menopause and vaginal infections may occur frequently.

MENOPAUSE

Menopause indicates the end of the menstrual cycles in a woman. It usually has its onset between the ages of 45 and 50 but may occur during the 40's in some women. There may be some symptoms which occur in women during menopause and this may be disturbing to the elderly females. Even though menopause, which is a natural phenomenon occurs in the 50's, it is discussed here as it is a sign of aging in women and is accompanied by variable symptoms.

What are the symptoms of menopause.

The symptoms of menopause occur due to the reduction in the natural female hormones in women. This occurs early in those women where the ovaries are removed during surgery or who have had radiation treatment.

- Initially, the monthly menstrual periods become irregular and occur at less frequent intervals before they completely stop.
- There may be dryness of the vagina.
- The woman may feel sudden feeling of warmth all over the body. These are called '**Hot Flashes**'. They may be accompanied by sweating.
- The hair may become thin and dry.
- The woman tends to put on weight.
- There may be mood changes in the woman with periods of depression.

Some of the effects of menopause in the woman may be the higher risk of developing heart disease and osteoporosis. The dryness of the vagina renders sexual activity painful. In some, urinary incontinence may occur as an after effect of menopause.

No specific tests are needed to diagnose menopause. Occasionally, the Gynecologist may order blood tests to assess the level of hormones.

Treatment.

Many women do not need treatment for menopausal symptoms. But when the symptoms are annoying enough, the doctor my prescribe hormones in small doses for the patient. *Estrogen* is the hormone given. In those with an intact uterus, it may be combined with another hormone named *Progesterone*.

The vaginal dryness and pain during sexual intercourse may be relieved with estrogen containing vaginal creams which are available. Over the counter lubricating creams for vaginal application are available.

In women in whom the hot flashes are troublesome, small doses of anti-depressant medication may be prescribed.

In addition, the woman will need medications for treating osteoporosis and urinary incontinence if they are present.

General Measures.

Some important general measures to control the symptoms of menopause are:

- Adequate exercise and good nutritious food. Foods containing calcium should be taken.
- In some women, the hot flashes are triggered by beverages like coffee or alcohol. Spicy food also may trigger hot flashes. It is wise to avoid them or limit their intake. A cool environment with air conditioning is helpful.
- Relaxation techniques like yoga, Tai-Chi and meditation are helpful in many women.
- Smoking should be avoided.
- The person should get enough sleep of at least 7 – 9 hours.
- When urinary incontinence is causing problems, pelvic floor exercises called *Kegels Exercises* (See below) are advised. (See section on Urinary Incontinence in Book 1).

PROLAPSE OF UTERUS

Uterine *prolapse* is a condition not uncommon in elderly women. As the woman gets older, the muscles and tissues in the pelvis which support the uterus weaken and the uterus begins to descend and ultimately protrude into the vagina. Many women who have had multiple deliveries may develop prolapse which is mild and often does not need treatment if the symptoms are absent or mild. But others may develop symptoms.

Symptoms of Prolapse of the Uterus.

- The patient feels a dragging feeling in the pelvis. This is often very uncomfortable. An aching feeling occurs in the low back.
- She feels a swelling coming down into the vagina. The uterus may be seen or felt as a bulge down in the vagina.
- Urinary symptoms like incontinence or a feeling of incomplete emptying of the bladder may be present. This is because, part of the urinary bladder is also dragged down along with the uterus.
- The patient may be constipated. This occurs as part of the rectum also prolapses.
- As the prolapse progresses, the woman may feel pain in the back and discomfort while sitting.
- Repeated urinary infections may occur in some women.
- Sexual intercourse often becomes painful.
- In severe cases of prolapse, the uterus may rub against the clothes and become infected and ulcerated.

What causes Prolapse of the Uterus.

A family history of prolapse, multiple childbirths, advanced age, and overweight are common causes.

Chronic asthma, and constipation can lead to the development of prolapse of the uterus because the pressure inside the abdomen increases when the woman coughs or strains when passing stools. This pushes the uterus down into the vagina through the weak pelvic floor.

Delivery of a large baby as in a diabetic woman can cause prolapse in old age. Difficult and prolonged delivery also can lead to prolapse later in life.

Smoking is a risk factor which can lead to prolapse of the uterus.

When symptoms as described above are present, the woman should consult a *Gynecologist*. The diagnosis is confirmed by the doctor after a thorough examination. Other tests may be needed if the patient has symptoms of urinary incontinence or severe prolapse.

How is prolapse of the uterus treated.

- When the prolapse is mild with few symptoms, **changes in one's lifestyle** can prevent further increase in the prolapse. The person should lose weight if obese. Constipation should be treated and straining avoided. Lifting of heavy weights should not be done.

- Some exercises are available to strengthen the muscles of the pelvic floor. They are regularly done to prevent further prolapse. These are called ***Kegels Exercises***. (See Section on *Urinary Incontinence in* Book 1).

- **Intrauterine *Pessaries*.** A *pessary* is a rubber or silicone device inserted into the uterus to support the uterus and prevent prolapse. This is useful only in mild cases of prolapse. They provide symptomatic relief in many patients and help control the urinary incontinence. But they have to be maintained properly with periodic cleaning and re-insertion. Complications like infection of the vagina may occur occasionally with pessaries. Pessaries are used in patients in whom surgery is not possible due to advanced age or other severe associated diseases.

- **Surgery** for prolapse of the uterus is the standard accepted treatment. Various types of surgical procedures are available. Repair of the pelvic floor muscles with strengthening is done in many cases. In some patients the uterus is removed surgically (*Hysterectomy*).

Can prolapse of the uterus be prevented.

Though damage done to the pelvic muscles or tissues during childbirth cannot be totally reversed to prevent prolapse, some methods are available by for prevention.

- Losing weight in overweight women is very important.

- Women should avoid lifting heavy weights.
- Constipation if present, should be appropriately treated with proper diet rich in fiber, fruits, and vegetables. Medications maybe needed.
- Smoking must be avoided. Chronic cough must be treated to prevent prolapse of the uterus.
- Regular exercises to strengthen the pelvic floor muscles should be done. (***Kegels Exercises***). In this the pelvic floor is tightened as if preventing passing stools or gas. This tightening is held for 5 – 10 seconds at a time and then relaxed. This is done about 10 – 15 times in one session. These exercises are repeated 3 or 4 times a day depending on the patient's convenience. The exercises can be done any time of the day and when sitting, watching TV, or lying down and is simple and convenient.

VULVOVAGINITIS

The *Vulva* is the part of the female genitals which is outside the body. They include the vaginal opening, urethral opening, the *clitoris,* and the rounded area above it covered with hair. Inflammation of the vulva and vagina is called *Vulvovaginitis*. This can be caused by bacteria or fungi.

Symptoms of Vulvovaginitis.

The main symptoms are felt in the vulva and the vagina of women.

- Itching may be present in the vulva and the vagina. Occasionally, a burning sensation is felt.
- Mild swelling of the vulva is often present.
- Pain or discomfort may be felt when passing urine and during sexual intercourse.
- A whitish, foul smelling discharge may occur from the vagina.
- Mild bleeding may occur in some patients.

A sample of the vaginal discharge can be examined in the laboratory to determine the cause of the infection.

Treatment.

Treatment depends on the cause of the infection. A fungal infection is treated using anti-fungal medications. These are given in the form of vaginal tablets which can be introduced into the vagina to act locally. Bacterial infections may need oral medications.

Prevention.

Cleanliness is most important in prevention. Perfumes and sprays should not be used on the vaginal or vulvar area. Tampons, if used should not be kept for more than 8 – 10 hours and changed frequently when they are soaked. Cotton undergarments should be worn and tight fitting clothes should be avoided. Douches should be avoided and condoms should be worn during sex by the male partner.

POST MENOPAUSAL BLEEDING

Menopause is the cessation of menstrual bleeding in a woman usually after the age of 45 or 50 years. It indicates that the ovaries have ceased to produce estrogen and do not produce eggs. Hence *menstruation* stops. <u>*A woman is said to have reached menopause if there is no menstrual bleeding for one year.*</u> In some women, there may be bleeding occurring in small quantities after they have attained menopause. This is called 'Post-Menopausal Bleeding' (**PMB**). It is abnormal and should be investigated without delay. Occasionally the bleeding is minimal and is called '*spotting*'.

What are the causes of Post-Menopausal Bleeding (PMB).

Post-menopausal bleeding should never be ignored as it may presage a serious disease. The common causes of PMB are:

- Atrophic Vaginitis where the vaginal lining is thinned out and inflamed causing it to bleed.
- There may be small non-cancerous growths inside the uterus or on the *cervix*. They are called '*Polyps*' and may bleed occasionally.
- Hormone Replacement Therapy (HRT) is a cause of PMB in some women as the hormones can cause menstrual like bleeding.
- Thinning of the *endometrium*, may lead to bleeding.
- Fibroids are non-cancerous tumors occurring in the uterus which may occasionally bleed in the post-menopausal woman. Even though fibroids tend to shrink after menopause, in some women it still causes bleeding.
- Occasionally the endometrium becomes very thick, a condition called Endometrial *Hyperplasia*, and this can lead to bleeding. When the endometrium thickens, some of the cells may become abnormal and later on may turn cancerous.

- The most dreaded cause of PMB is however, cancer which can be in the uterus or cervix.
- Sometimes, bleeding from adjacent structures like the urethra, bladder or the rectum may be mistaken for PMB.
- Certain medications like *anti-coagulants* (blood thinners) used for heart diseases may cause bleeding from the uterus.
- Sexual intercourse in some women may lead to bleeding as the vaginal inner lining is thin in the elderly and may bleed easily.

The diagnosis is by examination of the external genitals by a Gynecologist. The doctor examines the inside of the vagina and visualizes the cervix.

An Ultrasound examination of the uterus ovaries and other pelvic organs will be needed. This is done by introducing a small ultrasound probe into the vagina and performing the ultrasound examination.

A biopsy of the endometrium will be taken to diagnose the cause of the bleeding. If cancer or other changes in the cervix is suspected, a biopsy may be taken from the cervix.

Dilation & Curettage (**D&C**) is a test where a small instrument is passed into the uterus through the cervix and scrapings are taken from endometrium and sent for examination in the laboratory. This gives the details regarding the cells in the endometrium and whether cancer cells are present.

Hysteroscopy is a test where the Gynecologist looks inside the uterus using a small instrument with a camera at the tip. This gives the details of changes inside the uterus.

How is PMB treated.

The treatment depends on the cause of bleeding.

- When inflammation and infection are the causes, antibiotics are given.
- If thinning of the vaginal lining is due to low estrogen levels, estrogen may be given as oral tablets, vaginal creams, or

vaginal tablets.

- Small polyps are surgically removed.
- When fibroids are the reason for PMB, they should be removed surgically or by shrinking them by cutting off their blood supply through interventional procedures. Occasionally the whole uterus is removed.
- If cancer of the cervix or uterus is suspected, the treatment consists of removal of the uterus (*hysterectomy*) along with radiation therapy and chemotherapy.

CANCER OF THE FEMALE REPRODUCTIVE SYSTEM

Cancers of the sexual organs in women are of various types. They may affect the ovaries, uterus, cervix, vagina, or the vulva. All of these will be discussed here. Approximately 100,000 women are diagnosed with cancer of the female reproductive organs every year in the USA.

What are the Risk Factors for developing the Cancers.

- A virus named Human Papilloma Virus (HPV) which is transmitted by sexual intercourse is associated with the development of cancers of the vulva, uterus, and cervix in women. Hence the importance of practicing safe sex and the use of condoms.
- Smoking in the female can weaken the immunity of the patient and lead to a persistent infection with HPV.
- Age is an important factor. Women above the age of 60 have a higher risk of developing cancer.
- Obesity increases the risk of ovarian cancer.
- Family history of cancers of the reproductive system increases the chances of the cancer in a woman.
- The beginning of menstruation before the age of 12 in a girl or the delay in menopause in a women can be risk factors in the development of uterine cancer.
- Women who have not borne children have a higher risk of cancer of the uterus and ovaries.
- Women on hormone treatment run the risk of developing uterine and vaginal cancers.

What are the symptoms of Cancer of the Reproductive System.
The symptoms vary depending on the site of the cancer and how advanced it is. Some of the important symptoms are as follows.

- **Bleeding** from the vagina is the commonest symptom. This could be from the uterus, cervix or vagina depending on the site of origin of the cancer.
- **Cancer of the vulva** may be seen outside as an itchy wart-like growth. It can bleed on coming into contact with clothes or during sexual intercourse. Occasionally it may present as an *ulcer*.
- **Cancer of the vagina** is rare. Vaginal cancer may cause bleeding or a whitish discharge. A lump may be detected in the vagina Pain and difficulty in passing urine may be noticed.
- **Cancer of the cervix** may present with bleeding or a whitish discharge. Often the patient may notice bleeding after sexual intercourse. Intercourse may be painful. Dull aching pain in the pelvic region or cramps may occur.
- **Cancer of the uterus** may be of different types. Cancer of the *Endometrium* (lining of the uterus) is the commonest. It is one of the cancers that produces bleeding early in its course and hence is detected early. A post-menopausal woman with bleeding should be investigated for endometrial cancer. Pain in the pelvis and urinary symptoms may also occur.
- **Cancer of the ovaries** may not give any symptoms in early stages. There may be a feeling of bloating or urinary symptoms. Pelvic pain may be present in some patients. Urinary symptoms and constipation may be noted in others. Low back pain may occur.

Diagnosis.

Diagnosis depends on the site of the cancer. Various methods are adopted.

Cancer of the Vulva and Vagina can be detected by inspecting the area and examining the inside of the vagina. The Gynecologist will take a sample of the tissue (biopsy) and send it for laboratory examination.

<u>Cancer of the cervix</u> is diagnosed by inspecting the cervix with an instrument which magnifies the image. A biopsy or scrapings from the cervix may be taken for study.

<u>Cancer of the endometrium</u> is diagnosed using multiple methods. The Gynecologist examines the uterus through the vagina inserting two gloved fingers to feel the cervix and the uterus. An ultrasound examination of the uterus and adjoining structures can be done by inserting the probe of the instrument into the vagina (*Transvaginal Ultrasound*) and recording the images. The Gynecologist can see the inside of the uterus using an instrument with a camera and light at its tip. This is called the *Hysteroscope*. Multiple bits of tissue can be taken from the uterus to be examined in the laboratory. Occasionally, the Gynecologist may prefer to do a D&C to remove scrapings from the endometrium for laboratory study.

<u>Cancer of the ovary</u> may be detected by many methods. The Gynecologist performs the usual tests for feeling the uterus and ovaries through the vagina. A *Transvaginal ultrasound* is done to see the ovaries and the size of the tumor. A CT scan may be done to know the location, size, and other details of the cancer.

What are the modes of Treatment of Gynecological Cancers.

The treatment of the cancer will depend on the site of occurrence of the cancer and the extent of its spread. This is often determined by the Gynecologist in coordination with the *Oncologist*.

Cancer of the Vulva. Surgery is done to remove the cancer and part of the vulva. Occasionally, nearby lymph nodes are removed. Following this, Radiation therapy, Chemotherapy, Targeted Therapy, and Immunotherapy are used to treat the cancer.

Cancer of the Vagina. This is treated with surgery. Small tumors are removed directly. When it is larger, part, or whole of the vagina may be removed by the surgeon. Rarely the cervix and uterus are removed along with this. Following removal of the vagina, an artificial vagina is reconstructed using skin, intestine, or muscles from other parts of the body to form a new vagina which permits sexual intercourse.

Radiation therapy and Chemotherapy may be needed in some patients.

Cancer of the Cervix. When the cancer is its early stages, the affected part of the cervix is removed leaving the rest of the cervix and uterus intact. Occasionally, the whole cervix may be removed leaving the uterus in position. But when advanced, extensive surgery may be needed to remove the uterus and part of the vagina along with the lymph nodes. Often this is accompanied by additional Chemotherapy, Radiation, Targeted Therapy or Immunotherapy or a combination of these as the Gynecologists deems appropriate.

Cancer of the Uterus. The uterus, ovaries and the Fallopian tubes are removed surgically. Occasionally, the surrounding lymph nodes are removed. Chemotherapy, Radiation therapy, Immunotherapy, Hormone Therapy and Targeted therapy are occasionally offered for patients. Often, a combination of these is offered to the patient.

Cancer of the Ovary. Surgery in early stages may be done to remove the affected ovary. Both ovaries are removed if affected. In some cases, the uterus may have to be removed. In advanced cases, in addition, the lymph nodes in the pelvis are removed.

Chemotherapy, Immunotherapy and Targeted therapy are other methods of treatment. Chemotherapy may be occasionally given before and after surgery. Radiation therapy is given for ovarian cancer in some cases.

Palliative Care. Palliative care is the supportive care given to patients with advanced cancer (or any terminal illness) so as to improve their quality of life and make their remaining days as comfortable and painless as possible. This is done by a team of Palliative care providers who address the emotional, physical, social, and spiritual needs of the patients. The treatment for the underlying cancer continues even while the palliative care team addresses these concerns. The team provides solace to the patient in the final days. (See the chapter on *Palliative Therapy and End-of-Life Care.*)

Screening for Gynecological Cancers.

The screening for cancers of the female reproductive system is done in middle age.

Screening for cervical cancer is done to detect changes in the cells in the cervix before they become cancerous. These changes take about 3 – 7 years to become fully cancerous. The screening for cervical cancer is done in early adulthood, ideally starting at age 21 and is done once in 3 years up to the age of 65. Screening for cervical cancer is stopped after the age of 65. The doctor takes scapings from the cervix of the uterus and sends it for examination in the laboratory where these are examined for the presence of abnormal cells.

The Human Papilloma Virus is a cause of cervical cancer in women and hence, HPV vaccination is important to prevent this infection in women. HPV vaccination is given to children aged 11-12 years and is given 6-12 months apart as two injections. It can be given as early as 9 years. Though it is not given after the age of 26, adults above this age may take it in consultation with their Gynecologist.

Resources

1. Gynecological Assessment of the Elderly Patient. *Medscape.*

https://www.medscape.org/viewarticle/554398

1. Gynecological Disorders in the Older Patient. Jones JS, Montgomery M. *Academic Emergency Medicine.* 1994. 1 : 580-587

https://onlinelibrary.wiley.com/doi/pdf/10.1111/
j.1553-2712.1994.tb02560.x

1. General Information about Gynecological Cancer. *KSK Center of Irvine.*

https://kskcancercenter.com/conditions_gynecological

1. Endometrial Cancer. Overview. *Mayo Clinics*. 2021

https://www.mayoclinic.org/diseases-conditions/endometrial-cancer/symptoms-causes/syc-20352461

1. Post-Menopausal Bleeding. Sung S, Abramovitz A. *National Library of Medicine*. 2022

https://www.ncbi.nlm.nih.gov/books/NBK562188/

1. Vaginitis. *Hartford Healthcare. Senior Services* 2022
2. *https://hhcseniorservices.org/health-wellness/health-resources/health-library/detail?id=zx1776&lang=en-us*
3. Malignant Tumors of the Female Reproductive System. Weiderpass E, Labreche F. *Safety & Health At Work* 2012. 3 : pages 166-180

https://www.sciencedirect.com/science/article/pii/S2093791112330023?via%3Dihub

1. Updated Cervical Cancer Screening Guidelines. *American College of Obstetricians & Gynecologists*. 2021.

https://www.acog.org/clinical/clinical-guidance/practice-advisory/articles/2021/04/updated-cervical-cancer-screening-guidelines

10. HPV Vaccine. *Centers for Disease Control & Prevention*. 20212

https://www.cdc.gov/hpv/parents/vaccine-for-hpv.html#:~:text=HPV%20vaccination%20is%20not%20recommended,be
1.

---

1. https://www.cdc.gov/hpv/parents/vaccine-for-hpv.html#_853ae90f0351324bd73ea615e6487517__4c761f170e016836ff84498202b99827__853ae90f0351324bd73ea615e6487517_text_43ec3e5dee6e706af7766fffea512721_HPV_0bcef9c45bd8a48eda1b26eb0c61c869_20vaccination_0bcef9c45bd8a48eda1b26eb0c61c869_20is_0bcef9c45bd8a48eda1b26eb0c61c869_20not_0bcef9c45bd8a48eda1b26eb0c61c869_20recommended_c0cb5f0fcf239ab3d9c1fcd31fff1efc_benefits_0bcef9c45bd8a48eda1b26eb0c61c869_20of_0bcef9c45bd8a48eda1b26eb0c61c869_20vaccination_0bcef9c45bd8a48eda1b26eb0c61c869_20for_0bcef9c45bd8a48eda1b26eb0c61c869_20them

6. DISORDERS OF THE TEETH

Structure and Function. The teeth in humans have an important function of biting and chewing food. The teeth are needed for normal speech and pronunciation of words. They are one of the strongest structures in the human body, stronger than bones. A normal adult has 32 teeth. Of these 28 teeth erupt before the individual reaches age 14 and the last four teeth at the back of the jaws called "Wisdom teeth" erupt around the age of 18.

The part of the tooth seen above the gums is called the *Crown* and the part embedded in the jaw bone is called the *Root.*

The different parts of the teeth are described below. (**Figure 6**).

The **Enamel** is the part of the tooth that is seen outside the gums. It is the hardest substance in the human body and is formed of calcium phosphate which is a mineral as hard as a rock. It gives the enamel the bluish white color. The enamel has no blood supply or nerves.

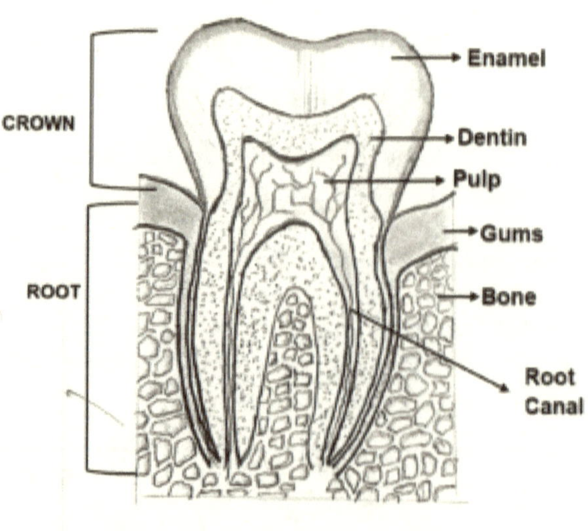

Figure 6

The **Dentin** is the part of the tooth beneath the enamel. This extends down the whole of the tooth. The dentin is not hard as the enamel and it is similar to bone. It is pale yellow in color.

The **Cementum** is the 'glue' that holds the tooth firmly in the bony socket of the jaw. It is composed of minerals and connective tissue and anchors the tooth firmly to the jaw bone. The **Pulp** is the inner core of the tooth inside the dentin. It contains soft cells along with blood vessels and nerves. The pulp supplies the tooth with nourishment. It is the exposed pulp which causes the tooth to be sensitive in tooth decay (*Caries*). The root of the tooth thus consists of dentin, pulp, and cementum. The exposed area above the gums (Crown) consists of the enamel and the dentin beneath it.

Dental problems in old age are common. As one ages, the tissues in the body become thinner and less elastic. The multiplication of cells is slower. Bones become less dense and strong. All these changes affect the teeth too, leading to loose teeth and decay. The color of the teeth tends to become yellow with age as the dentin is seen through. The enamel may wear off in old age due to constant usage. Chipping of the enamel may occur in old age.

As a person grows old, cell multiplication slows down, the immunity wanes, tissues tend to become thinner and lose their elasticity, and the density and strength of the bones become less. The jaw bones which anchor the teeth become weaker, the tissues that hold the teeth in their sockets become thinner and less elastic leading to loose teeth and erosion. Furthermore, the secretion of saliva by the salivary glands decreases with age leading to various dental problems.

For an elderly individual with his front teeth missing, speech becomes difficult and he is not able to pronounce certain words correctly. When the teeth on the sides are missing, chewing becomes difficult. Often this leads to poor nutrition and depression as they find it embarrassing to interact with other individuals in society. Similarly, the teeth are worn due to constant use and teeth-grinding which occurs in some individuals. The height of the tooth is reduced and the enamel of the tooth gets worn off.

Some of the common dental problems seen in old age are Dryness of the mouth, Gum disease, Cavities, Caries, Bad Breath, and Mouth Cancer.

DRY MOUTH

Dryness of the mouth called *Xerostomia* in medical parlance, is very common in old age. About 30% of individuals above the age of 65 and 40% of those above 80 have dry mouth. Dry mouth is found to be common in those taking more than four or more types of medications for various systemic diseases.

Normally saliva secreted by the salivary glands lubricates the mouth and helps to maintain overall oral health. Saliva is necessary for appreciating the taste of food. It helps in protecting tooth decay and keeping the gums healthy. Saliva has the mild ability to kill bacteria. It helps in chewing and swallowing by wetting the food. Dryness of mouth makes it difficult for the elderly person to chew and swallow dry foods like bread, *chapati* and dry salads.

As a person ages, the saliva production by the salivary glands decreases. In addition, diseases like diabetes, alcoholic cirrhosis, rheumatoid arthritis, stress, and anxiety can produce a dry mouth. Medications like those used for high blood pressure, depression, and certain neurological diseases may cause a dry mouth.

Treatment of dry mouth aims at finding the offending causes and treating them.

- Diseases like diabetes should be kept under control.
- Medications causing a dry mouth may be changed in consultation with one's doctor.
- Tobacco products which increase dryness of the mouth should be avoided.
- Frequent drinking of warm water is beneficial.
- While eating food, frequent sips of water or any liquid is advisable to make chewing easier. Foods which are dry like cookies, dry bread or rusk may be soaked in a liquid like milk or coffee and eaten.

- Sucking on sugar free candies or sugar free chewing gum helps in increasing saliva flow.
- Mouthwashes and saliva substitutes are available for dry mouth.
- Mouth breathing should be avoided. Nasal problems should be adequately treated.
- A humidifier in the room helps to reduce dryness of the mouth.

TOOTH DECAY

Tooth decay also called *Dental Caries*, leads to infection pain and ultimately, to loss of teeth. Dryness of mouth and an increased intake of sweets and sugars are often causative. Sugar and starch containing food particles in the mouth are broken down by the bacteria in the mouth to acids which corrode the hard surfaces of the teeth to form cavities. When the cavities are deep, the nerves in the pulp of the tooth are exposed and this leads to sensitivity and pain.

Dental caries often leads to infection of the root of the tooth resulting in pain and inflammation. Occasionally it is severe causing swelling and extreme pain. It affects the quality of life of the individual. It has been noted that dental caries peaks in three ages of life – 6, 25 and 70 years. The elderly, hence, are at an increased risk of developing tooth decay.

In the elderly, there may be gum disease which leads to recession of the gums which causes the roots of the teeth to be exposed. This may lead to decay of the root causing infection and falling or breaking of the tooth.

Dental caries is seen commonly in those who have poor oral hygiene, use tobacco, chew betel nuts, and belong to the lower socioeconomic strata of society. Other causes of caries are dryness of mouth, excess consumption of sugar containing foods or beverages, decrease in saliva, previous history of caries in young age, Those who do not use toothpaste containing fluoride are prone to dental caries.

Plaque and *Tartar* build up in the teeth when brushing and cleaning of the teeth are improper. A *plaque* is a sticky coating of bacteria which forms on the surface of the teeth. *Tartar* is a hard deposit containing calcium which forms on the surface of the teeth if the plaques are not removed by regular brushing. Once the tartar forms, it is not easy to remove them. They must be removed by the dentist or the dental hygienist.

How is Dental Caries treated.

Fluoride treatment is given for patients with dental caries. This is done by the dental surgeon and is useful in early cases of caries.

In more advanced cases, the cavities may be filled using various materials.

When the enamel has been destroyed, the dental surgeon replaces the crown with an artificial material like porcelain, resin, or metal.

When the cavity is deeper affecting the pulp, 'Root Canal Treatment' is offered, where the pulp is removed and a filling put in. This is followed by replacing the crown with artificial material.

When the cavity is very deep and the tooth cannot be salvaged, it is extracted by the dental surgeon.

GUM DISEASE

Disease of the gums is called **Periodontitis**. It has been reported that two out of three persons above the age of 65 have disease of the gums. Infection of the gums is not uncommon in old age. This is a consequence of poor oral hygiene and lack of regular brushing of teeth. The gums often recede in old age exposing the roots. The roots thus exposed may decay and get infected ultimately leading to loss of the teeth.

Infection and inflammation of the gums can lead to loss of teeth. Gum inflammation is called *Gingivitis* and is an important risk factor for heart disease. Smoking, diabetes, and a weak immune system as in the elderly are causes for development of gum disease. Untreated gum disease is often associated with aggravation of diabetes and treating the gum disease often gives a better control of diabetes.

Gum disease is treated by removing the plaques and tartar by the dental surgeon or hygienist. Antibiotics are needed if there is bacterial infection. Various type of dental surgical treatments are available for the treatment of gum disease.

ORAL CANCER

Cancer of the mouth is called 'Oral Cancer'. It is twice as common in men compared to women. In the US in 2022, approximately 54,000 cases of oral cancer are expected to occur. Mouth cancer usually occurs above the age of 60 but may occur at a younger age.

The site of occurrence of the cancer may be the tongue, inner aspect of the cheeks, gums, roof of the mouth (palate), lips, salivary glands, and throat. The type of cancer may vary depending on where it occurs.

What are the symptoms of Oral Cancer.

Oral cancer may present in various ways. Often in the early stages, it may go undetected and is easily missed except when a dental surgeon or a hygienist examines the mouth.

- A non-healing mouth ulcer may be cancerous. If a mouth ulcer persists for more than two or three weeks, it should be examined by a dental surgeon to rule out the possibility of cancer.
- Swellings or growths occurring inside the mouth, side of the tongue, inner aspect of the cheek, gums, or the presence of large lymph nodes in the neck of the patient may indicate a cancer.
- Occasionally, whitish, or reddish patches may be seen in the mouth in the inner aspect of the cheeks or tongue. They may indicate a pre-cancerous condition and should be examined by a dental surgeon.
- Occasionally these lumps or ulcers may bleed to touch, while eating food or brushing the teeth. Any bleeding from the mouth should alert one to consult the dental surgeon.
- A numb feeling in the tongue or lips may be a symptom of cancer in some.
- If the area of a tooth extraction does not heal, but continues

to bleed, oral cancer should be suspected.

- When the cancer is at the back of the mouth, difficulty in moving the jaw and opening the mouth may be present.
- Cancer of the throat interferes with swallowing and speech. It may lead to pain during swallowing.

What are the common causes of Oral Cancer.

- **Tobacco** use in any form is dangerous and can lead to oral cancer. Cigarettes, cigars, and pipe smoking are important causes. Tobacco is used in the South Asian countries for chewing and the quid is kept in the mouth for long periods. This is an important cause of cancer in countries like India, Pakistan, and other Asian countries.
- **Alcohol** consumption can cause of oral cancer. Cancer of the mouth and throat is seen in heavy drinkers. It is found that drinking alcohol along with smoking poses the highest risk. The risk for oral cancer is 30 times more for a person who drinks and smokes compared to one who neither smokes nor drinks alcohol.
- **Betel nut chewing** is a cause of cancer in the South Asian countries. Often the betel nut is chewed along with betel leaves and tobacco and kept in the mouth as a quid for long periods.
- **Human Papilloma Virus infection** (HPV) is important in the causation of oral cancer. It is often transmitted by sexual contact and is a cause of cancer in the mouth and throat. In addition, HPV can cause cancer of the cervix, vagina, penis, and anus.
- **Poor oral hygiene** is an important risk factor in the development of mouth cancer. The presence of sharp teeth or ill-fitting dentures can cause ulcers on the cheeks or tongue due to constant irritation leading to cancer.

- **Over exposure to sunlight** is a cause of cancer of the lips. People who work outdoors for prolonged periods are at a higher risk.
- **Poor nutrition** and an unhealthy diet have been cited as a cause for oral cancer.

How is mouth cancer diagnosed.

A *biopsy* of the lesion gives the diagnosis. A small bit of tissue is removed under local anesthesia and sent to the laboratory for studies. The cancer can be confirmed by this and the type of cell causing the cancer identified.

Further investigations like X-rays, CT scan, MRI scan or PET scan are usually needed only when contiguous spread to nearby structures or remote structures like the lung, liver or brain is suspected in advanced cancer.

How is mouth cancer treated.

The treatment of the cancer of the mouth depends on the stage of the cancer and whether it has spread to other structures.

In early stages, when the cancer is confined to the mouth, it can be easily removed by surgery. The type of surgery will depend on its location. Cancer of the tongue may need removal of part of the tongue. If it is in the cheek, that part of the cheek is removed and later plastic surgery is done to cover up the gap. If the cancer is attached to the jaw, then part of the jaw has is removed. Often the surgery is followed by plastic surgery to reconstruct the area using skin, muscle, and bone from other parts of the body of the patient.

Chemotherapy, Radiation therapy, and Immunotherapy are used either in conjunction with surgery or after surgery according to the extent of involvement of the cancer.

Brachytherapy is a form of radiation treatment where radioactive implants are placed directly inside the tumor and left in place for variable periods of 1 – 8 days. They may be in the form of small needles or pellets. They are then removed. This type of radiation treatment is called 'Internal Radiation' compared to conventional Radiation Therapy which is called External Radiation'.

Complications of mouth cancer

Difficulty in swallowing is the most important complication which can occur in cancers of the back of the mouth and throat. Cancer of the tongue interferes with eating.

Difficulty in speech often results from large growths in the mouth as they cause difficulty in articulation.

Cancer of the mouth, since it interferes with feeding of the patient, leads to nutritional problems and malnutrition.

Psychological problems like depression are very commonly associated with cancers of the mouth.

Complications may occur following treatment. Radiation therapy may lead to dryness of the mouth and difficulty in swallowing. Disfigurement of the face is often present following surgery, even though it can be corrected to a large extent by reconstructive plastic surgery. Infection in the mouth, ulceration, bleeding, tooth decay and loss of teeth are other complications which may occur following treatment.

The treatment of mouth cancer is a team work which includes the cancer surgeon, the dental surgeon, the plastic surgeon, and the Oncologist. Often the patient may need psychotherapy support following surgery for the emotional and psychological trauma.

Prevention Of Dental Problems In Old Age.

This is discussed under a separate head as the preventive measures mentioned here are common to all the diseases discussed above.

- Smoking and tobacco use in any form is taboo.
- Alcohol consumption should be moderate as recommended – not more than two drinks of hard liquor a day for men and one for women.
- Excess sugary foods and snacks should be avoided. The mouth should be rinsed with water every time a sugary drink or snack

is taken. This prevents dental caries and cavities. Acid is present in citrus juices, fizzy drinks, and many juices. The mouth should be rinsed with water after taking these drinks. Milk or cheese taken after these drinks can 'neutralize' their effect to some extent.

- Chewing on sugarless or xylitol containing chewing gum can promote flow of saliva and prevent problems of dry mouth.

- The teeth should be brushed twice daily using a toothpaste containing fluoride. Fluoride mouth rinses or fluoride varnishes applied to the teeth may be needed on the advice of the dental surgeon. The teeth should be brushed after every meal to prevent plaque and tartar formation.

- The teeth should be flossed at least once daily using dental floss. The elderly may be given floss holders for convenience of usage.

- A firm toothbrush should be used. Ideally, it should be changed every three months. Electric toothbrushes are useful for those elderly who have arthritis and difficulty in holding the toothbrushes.

- Wear and tear on teeth and chipping of the enamel can be prevented by avoiding very hard foods or using the teeth to open bottle caps. If the teeth are chipped or broken, prompt attention of a dental surgeon is called for.

- Those having dentures should keep them clean. Dentures should be placed in water every night while retiring. An appropriate cleaner may be used as advised by the dental hygienist.

- Antiseptic mouthwashes should be used after consulting the dental hygienist or the dental surgeon.

- A visit to the dental surgeon twice a year is ideal to keep the teeth and gums healthy and to detect any problems early. Six-monthly inspection of the mouth for any ulcers or lumps is important. The presence of sharp teeth or ill-fitting dentures should be managed at the earliest.

- The dental surgeon should be informed about any systemic disease that the patient has and the medications being taken.
- The presence of any prosthetic heart valves, pacemakers, artificial joints, or other implants should be informed to the dental surgeon as antibiotic *prophylaxis* must be given before doing any dental procedures on the patient.

Resources

1.   Aging changes in Teeth and Gums. Dugdale DC. *Medline Plus* 2022.

https://medlineplus.gov/ency/patientinstructions/000951.htm

1.   Common Oral conditions in Older patients. *American Family Physician* 2008

https://www.aafp.org/pubs/afp/issues/2008/1001/p845.html

1.   Common Medical and Dental Problems of Older Adults. A Narrative Review. Ying Chan AK et al. *Geriatrics* 2021. 6: page 76.

https://www.ncbi.nlm.nih.gov/pmc/articles/PMC8395714/

1.   Older Adult Oral Health. *Centers for Disease Control & Prevention* 2021.

https://www.cdc.gov/oralhealth/basics/adult-oral-health/
adult_older.htm#:~:text=About%202%20in%203%20(68,or%20older%20have%
[1]).

1.   Aging and Dental Health. *American Dental Association.* 2021.

https://www.ada.org/resources/research/science-and-research-institute/
oral-health-topics/aging-and-dental-
health#:~:text=Dental%20conditions%20associated%20with%20aging,including
[2].

1.   Aging Changes in Teeth and Gums. *Medline Plus.* National Library of
     Medicine. 2022

https://medlineplus.gov/ency/patientinstructions/000951.htm

1.   Mouth Cancer – Overview - *NHS Website.* 2022 https://www.nhs.uk/
     conditions/mouth-cancer/

---

1. https://www.cdc.gov/oralhealth/basics/adult-oral-health/
adult_older.htm#_853ae90f0351324bd73ea615e6487517__4c761f170e016836ff84498202b99827__853ae90f03
51324bd73ea615e6487517_text_43ec3e5dee6e706af7766fffea512721_About_0bcef9c45bd8a48eda1b26eb0c61c
869_202_0bcef9c45bd8a48eda1b26eb0c61c869_20in_0bcef9c45bd8a48eda1b26eb0c61c869_203_0bcef9c45bd
8a48eda1b26eb0c61c869_20_84c40473414caf2ed4a7b1283e48bbf4_68_c0cb5f0fcf239ab3d9c1fcd31fff1efc_or_
0bcef9c45bd8a48eda1b26eb0c61c869_20older_0bcef9c45bd8a48eda1b26eb0c61c869_20have_0bcef9c45bd8a48
eda1b26eb0c61c869_20gum_0bcef9c45bd8a48eda1b26eb0c61c869_20disease._6cff047854f19ac2aa52aac51bf3a
f4a_text_43ec3e5dee6e706af7766fffea512721_Tooth_0bcef9c45bd8a48eda1b26eb0c61c869_20loss._c0cb5f0fcf2
39ab3d9c1fcd31fff1efc_65_0bcef9c45bd8a48eda1b26eb0c61c869_2D74_0bcef9c45bd8a48eda1b26eb0c61c869
_20_84c40473414caf2ed4a7b1283e48bbf4_13_0bcef9c45bd8a48eda1b26eb0c61c869_25

2. https://www.ada.org/resources/research/science-and-research-institute/oral-health-topics/aging-and-dental-
health#_853ae90f0351324bd73ea615e6487517__4c761f170e016836ff84498202b99827__853ae90f0351324bd7
3ea615e6487517_text_43ec3e5dee6e706af7766fffea512721_Dental_0bcef9c45bd8a48eda1b26eb0c61c869_20co
nditions_0bcef9c45bd8a48eda1b26eb0c61c869_20associated_0bcef9c45bd8a48eda1b26eb0c61c869_20with_0b
cef9c45bd8a48eda1b26eb0c61c869_20aging_c0cb5f0fcf239ab3d9c1fcd31fff1efc_including_0bcef9c45bd8a48eda
1b26eb0c61c869_20local_0bcef9c45bd8a48eda1b26eb0c61c869_20anesthetics_0bcef9c45bd8a48eda1b26eb0c6
1c869_20and_0bcef9c45bd8a48eda1b26eb0c61c869_20analgesics

7. PSYCHOLOGICAL DISORDERS

Psychological illness is often seen in elderly persons. But it may go unnoticed as it is often considered a part of the 'normal' aging process. It is often the close relatives of the elderly individual who notice these changes first. **Health issues, social isolation** and **cognitive decline** are the three main factors which can lead to psychological problems in old age. It is found that approximately 15% of the elderly individuals above the age of 60 have some mental problems.(World Health Organization).

Some of the reasons why the elderly develop mental problems can be summarized as:

- <u>Social isolation</u> is a common cause in the elderly. In the western society, the elderly live alone isolated from their kith and kin. The children once grown up leave the nest to fend for themselves. This is not commonly seen in many Asian countries like India and China where the elderly are cared for by the families and their children.

- <u>Cognitive decline</u> occurs to some extent with old age and their mental abilities are not sharp as when they were young. The recognition of their own helplessness can lead to problems like depression.

- <u>Physical health problems</u> like heart disease, diabetes and diseases of the joints and muscles may limit their movements and their ability to look after themselves. This may lead to dependency on others which affects their mental health.

- <u>Losing one's partner</u> can not only cause a feeling of loneliness and helplessness, but it also leads to depression and other psychological problems.

- <u>Malnourishment,</u> due to many factors is not uncommon in the elderly and this can add to the mental problems.

- <u>Multiple medications</u> and their side effects may cause a change in their mood and behaviour.

Some of the common disorders in old age are Memory Loss, Alzheimer's Disease, Delusion and Confusional States, Depression, Anxiety, Substance abuse, Bipolar disorder, and Schizophrenia. Of these, **Delusion & Confusional States, Memory Loss, and Alzheimer's Disease** have been discussed in detail in Book 1 of the series under the *Disorders of the Brain and Nervous System* and hence will not be dealt with here. (Ref: *How to Face the Health Challenges While Growing Old- Book 1*)

There are some risk factors which may be instrumental in the causation of mental illness in old age.

- <u>Retirement</u> of an individual from an active profession or job can lead to mental depression in the person as he feels suddenly cut off from his familiar surroundings in his office and feels that there is '*nothing else to do*'. After retirement, many individuals feel a sense of dependency on others and an apparent loss of self-respect. They also feel that they have lost their authority over others including family members and this could lead to depression or anxiety.

- <u>Nuclear Families,</u> where the elderly are left to fend for themselves can lead to various mental problems like anxiety and depression. In Asian countries like India, where usually, the parents live with their children even after the sons and daughters are married, psychological changes may occur when the children have to leave the parents due to their occupation or profession. Many children opt to go abroad to seek greener pastures and settle there leaving the aged parents behind. When the aged parent retires from an active job, he feels a sense of helplessness and loneliness if his children are not with him.

- <u>Income</u> of the elderly is low as they are no more employed. This leads to a change in their lifestyle and a feeling of dependency on their children and others which may lead to mental problems.

DEPRESSION

Depression affects almost 6 million Americans over the age of 65. It is said to be present in about 5% of the elderly individuals. Mild depression in the elderly may often go unnoticed or ignored as the symptoms are attributed to aging alone.

What are the common causes of Depression in the Elderly.

The common causes of depression in the elderly population are:

- <u>Physical health problems</u> like Heart disease, Stroke, Parkinson's disease, cancer, arthritis, and many other debilitating chronic diseases of old age.
- <u>Loneliness and social isolation</u> giving the person a feeling of desolation and helplessness can lead eventually to depression in an elderly individual.
- <u>Stress</u> due to any reason may present with depression. It could be due to financial reasons, social reasons, or health issues.
- <u>Exercise</u> is one way to keep up one's spirits and is an antidote to depression. The elderly may not exercise either due to physical inability or due to inertia. This can lead to a sedentary existence where the person sinks into a depressive state.
- <u>Sleep problems</u> like insomnia could lead to depression.
- <u>Substance abuse</u> or <u>alcohol addiction</u> may be an important cause of depression which is likely to be overlooked in the elderly living alone.
- A <u>family history of depression</u> may be a factor in old age depression.
- <u>Women</u> are more prone to depression. Being single, unmarried, divorced or widowed, increases the chances of depression

Symptoms of Depression.

The symptoms of depression in the elderly may be different from the depression seen in the young. *The caregiver and relatives should bear in mind that the symptoms of a serious underlying physical illness may mimic depression and hence medical problems should be excluded before the patient is diagnosed with depression.*

- An elderly person constantly feeling tired or 'exhausted' in the absence of a significant physical illness may be depressed.
- Communication may be reduced and the elderly may tend to become more silent and fail to express their feelings when they are depressed. This may be misconstrued by the relatives as obstinacy or arrogance. They may speak slowly or with a low voice. They appear to be withdrawn.
- A feeling of sorrow, helplessness or desolation is a common symptom of depression. In the elderly, however, the 'sadness' may not be present but may be expressed as 'lack of interest' in activities which used to interest them previously. All pleasurable activities including sex may be shunned by the individual.
- Sleeplessness or *Insomnia* is often a symptom of depression in many elderly individuals. They awake very early in the morning and are not able to fall asleep after waking. In some, excess sleep is a sign of depression.
- The person may complain of pain *"all over the body"*, not confined to any specific area or site. No physical cause for the pain, however, is found on examination.
- The elderly person with depression often finds it difficult to concentrate on a job or while reading. They have difficulty in making decisions and often depend on others to do so.
- Some patients with depression may be irritable and have difficulty in sitting still. Fidgeting is often a sign in depression.
- Entertaining thoughts of death or suicide is not rare in these individuals.

- One should remember that the expression of symptoms of depression may vary depending on the cultural background of the individual.

How to treat Depression in the Elderly.

One of the important aspects of treatment of depression is finding out if there is a physical illness like heart disease, diabetes, nervous system disease or any other illness causing the depression. This can be ascertained by proper history and physical examination of the patient by a physician. Physical illnesses, if present, should be optimally controlled. The various modalities of managing depression in the elderly are discussed below.

Counseling or Psychotherapy. The elderly individual is interviewed by a Psychologist or a Psychiatrist and is given a patient listening. The type of psychotherapy depends on factors like the cultural background of the patient, his education, previous employment, presence of cognitive dysfunction and the risk of suicide. In addition to this, active emotional support from family members and friends is very important in managing a person with depression.

Medications. Various medications are available in the treatment of depression and the Psychiatrist chooses the medication depending on the type of depression and presence of other co-morbidities. The side effects of all medications must be considered when prescribing them for patients with depression. The relatives and caregiver should be warned of these side effects and advised to be on the lookout for them.

Other Treatment modalities. These are *Electroconvulsive Therapy* (ECT), where a mild electric shock is given to the brain by placing electrodes on the scalp. Another method is *Repetitive Transcranial Magnetic Stimulation* where magnets are placed on the scalp to activate the brain.

How can Depression be prevented in the Elderly.

Though depression due to physical ailments may not be prevented, there are some factors which should be addressed.

- <u>Regular physical exercise</u> helps to elevate the mood in individuals. exercise increases the chemicals called Endorphins released from the brain and these are the *'feel-good'* chemicals which boost the mood of the individual. Further, exercise relieves stress to a great extent and functions as an antidote to depression.

- <u>A healthy diet</u> which is adequate in nutrients and calories is essential to maintain the physical health of the elderly individual. At the same time, the person should be careful not to put on excess weight.

- <u>Sleep</u> is essential in the prevention. At least 7 -9 hours of sleep is necessary for good mental health in old age.

- <u>Social activities</u> should be encouraged whenever possible. In olden days, the concept of a joint family system, especially in Asian countries was an ideal recipe for preventing depression in old age. The presence of children and grandchildren in the family, kept the elderly active and engaged, thus preventing thoughts of depression. The elder members of the family transferred the cultural legacies of their generation to the children and taught them the values and morals in life. Their experiences and knowledge could be shared with the younger generation. Sadly, this engagement of the elderly population is lacking in the modern society and depression tends to increase in such situations.

- <u>Enjoyable activities and games</u> which help prevent thoughts of loneliness and depression should be encouraged.

- <u>Activities at home</u> make them feel 'wanted' in the family. Local outings and picnics for the elderly, taking them out to the park, to visit music concerts and taking them along while visiting friends and attending social gatherings will keep loneliness away.

- <u>Picnics and excursions</u> avoid the monotony of daily living and give them time to express themselves. This should particularly be encouraged in those who live in institutions.

- <u>Pets</u> provide relief to the elderly preventing depression in them.

- <u>Spirituality</u> is a great way to ward off depression in the elderly. Depending on one's religious inclination, the elderly can be encouraged to attend religious discourses, *Bhajans*, *Satsangs*, prayer group meetings, sermons, and visit places of worship where they can interact with members of their age group. Going on pilgrimages to remote places of worship has been a time-tested way of keeping the elderly engaged and free of mental symptoms in countries like India.

ANXIETY

Next to depression, anxiety is the most common mental disorder in the elderly. WHO reports that approximately 3.8% of the elderly have anxiety. Anxiety disorders are poorly recognized and under treated. There are many types of anxiety disorders and they are mentioned below. Studies from India reveal them to be present in 10.8% of the elderly population.

Types of Anxiety Disorders.

<u>Generalized Anxiety Disorder</u>. (**GAD**) In this type of disorder the person worries about many things. There is no particular cause for worry. They worry and become anxious regarding every life situation even though they are aware that their anxiety is 'unnecessary'. They fear that the worst will happen to them in a given situation.

<u>Phobias</u>. In this type of anxiety disorder, the person has a specific fear of something or some situation. Examples are fear of heights (Agoraphobia), fear of closed spaces (Claustrophobia), fear of insects (Entomophobia), fear of fire (Pyrophobia) and so on.

<u>Panic Disorder.</u> Here, the person feels sudden severe attacks of anxiety or panic without any apparent reason. The person is terrified. The individual feels chest pain, sweating, palpitations, abdominal cramps, dizziness and feels as if he is going to die. Often the person goes to the physician thinking that he has a 'heart attack'.

<u>Obsessive Compulsive Disorder.</u> (**OCD**) These patients have recurrent thoughts that keeps nagging their mind. This is called *'Obsession'*. They feel compelled to repeat the same process -*'Compulsion'*. This may lead to doing the same act repeatedly as washing one's hands, checking the door to see if it is locked, cleaning repeatedly, compulsive counting, keeping things in order repeatedly, checking if the gas stove is switched off and so on.

<u>Post-Traumatic Stress Disorder.</u> (**PTSD**) After a major traumatic event in a person, the person may feel symptoms of anxiety repeatedly.

The event may be a natural disaster like floods, earthquake or hurricane, manmade disasters like a bomb blast, fire, accident, violence, physical abuse, or war. They may have nightmares, flashbacks, depression, sudden bouts of anxiety, sleep disorders, being startled easily, irritability and trouble concentrating.

What causes Anxiety in Elderly Individuals.

The common causes or Risk Factors for developing anxiety in an elderly individual are:

- Death of a loved one (spouse) leading to a feeling of isolation, loneliness, and helplessness.
- Sudden loss of independence when one retires and feels dependent on others.
- Financial worries.
- Anxiety may be caused due to the side effects of certain medications like steroids, asthma medications, caffeine preparations, thyroid medicines and some medicines used for nervous system disorders.
- Systemic diseases like heart disease, stroke, diabetes, or arthritis which limit one's day to day activities.
- Sleep disturbances, mainly insomnia.
- Alcohol or other substance abuse can lead to anxiety disorder.

How is anxiety in old age treated.

Some of the methods of treating anxiety in the elderly are:

- Psychotherapy or counseling is the usual method of tackling anxiety in old age. The help of a psychologist or psychotherapist is sought. They talk to the patient and get them to understand their fears and anxiety.
- "Exposure Therapy" or "Desensitization Therapy" is a type of treatment where the patient is exposed to the cause of his fear in a graded manner and gradually learns to overcome the fear.

This is useful in treating phobias.

- In many elderly individuals, Relaxation therapy in the form of Yoga and Mindfulness Meditation are useful in relieving anxiety.

- Art therapy, Music therapy, and Dance therapy are others forms of therapy practiced for anxiety.

- Physical exercise helps to reduce stress and anxiety in many individuals. Aerobic exercises like walking, swimming, and cycling are helpful if the physical condition of the elderly individual permits it. The elderly should be encouraged to go outdoors and walk in parks or gardens and not remain home bound. Exercise stimulates blood flow to the brain and stimulates the overall metabolism of the individual and has a positive effect on mood.

- Socializing is an important aspect of managing anxiety in the elderly. They should be encouraged to involve in social activities, partake in group activities for senior citizens and attend senior citizen clubs, day care centers for senior citizens, *Satsangs*, and reading clubs.

- Having, routine sleep habits like going to bed and awakening at regular times and getting 7 – 9 hours of sleep at night help to relieve the symptoms of anxiety.

- All co-existing medical illnesses should be adequately treated to give maximum relief to the patient from pain or other symptoms.

- Avoiding alcohol, smoking and other drug usage should be advised to rid the patient of anxiety.

- Taking a good nutritional diet is of paramount importance. Caffeine containing beverages must be reduced.

- Medications are available for treatment of anxiety and are prescribed by the physician when needed. Panic attacks may need emergency care. Occasionally anti-depressant medications are given to the patient when anxiety co exists with depression.

It must be remembered that the elderly are very sensitive people who have faced the 'slings and arrows' of life and are at the threshold of their sunset years. They have to be handled delicately and cared for by the near and dear ones and caregivers. They should be spoken to in a gentle manner. One should never be harsh or rude to them. It must be remembered that the elderly leave footprints on the sands of time for the younger generation to follow.

BIPOLAR DISORDER

Bipolar disorder is a disorder of mood where the patient exhibits alternative mood swings of elation and depression. Even though the disorder may have its onset in adolescence or early adulthood, bipolar disorder may occur after the age of 50 in some individuals. The onset of symptoms of mania in the elderly should make the physician think of other neurological diseases like stroke or dementia.

What are the causes of Bipolar Disorder in the Elderly.

A few causes for the development of this disorder in the elderly individuals are:

- Some individuals have dementia preceding the bipolar disorder and causing it.
- Patients with stroke may develop bipolar disorder following the neurological illness.
- There are certain rare diseases of the nervous system where specific areas of the brain are damaged leading to symptoms of bipolar disorder.
- Genes play a role in the genesis of bipolar disorder and it may run in families.

What are the symptoms of the disorder.

The symptoms encountered in patients with the disorder varies depending on the phase of the disease.

The symptoms during the <u>Depressive phase</u> are:

- Sleep may be disturbed causing excess somnolence.
- Some patients have thoughts of suicide.
- They constantly feel sad and have a low self-esteem and a feeling of hopelessness.
- The patient neglects to take care of himself and ignores

grooming and cleaning. The patient loses interest in all activities and is not able to enjoy when others around him are immersed in revelry.

- Social withdrawal, confusion, and difficulty in taking decisions is often present.
- They lose self-respect and may cry without a reason.
- They have difficulty in concentrating and cannot focus on a single job.
- They tend to depend on others for even minor things which they could do independently previously.
- They may complain of aches and pains in the body without any obvious cause.
- Their memory is impaired, they are confused and often disoriented.

The symptoms during the <u>Maniac phase</u> are:

- They seem over energetic and irritable. They may be euphoric and aggressive.
- They may have delusions.
- They are overtalkative and often talk irrelevantly.

- Some patients may exhibit risky behavior like driving fast, gambling away money, spending money lavishly without any reason etc. They may give away their possessions without thinking of the consequences, indulge in risky sexual behavior or invest unwisely.
- Insomnia is often present in the maniac phase.
- They may have feelings of grandeur and inflated self-esteem thinking highly of themselves and demand respect from others.

In between the manic and the depressed phase of bipolar disorder, there may be a variable period during which the person may appear totally normal with normal mood and behaviour.

Treatment of Bipolar Disorder.

Treatment of this condition consists of two parts – Medications and Psychotherapy.

Medications for Bipolar Disorder. Various types of medications are available for the treatment and they can be obtained only on the prescription of a qualified Psychiatrist. Certain special considerations are needed in the elderly while treating them in view of their age and metabolism.

- The elderly metabolize the medications slowly compared to younger individuals.
- The elderly are more sensitive to the effect of drugs used in this disorder. Hence low doses may suffice.
- Side effects of the drugs like dizziness and *vertigo* are more common in the elderly. This may lead to complications like falls and injury.
- Sedation due to the drugs is more pronounced in the elderly and this may interfere with their daily activities like eating or self-care.
- As the elderly are often on other medications for systemic illnesses like heart disease, diabetes or hypertension, interaction among these medications can lead to various adverse effects.

Psychotherapy. Psychotherapy by a qualified counselor is part of the treatment of bipolar disorder. Various methods are adopted in psychotherapy including counseling, family therapy, group therapy and ways to cope with stress which is a trigger for episodes of depression or mania. Often the combination of psychotherapy with medications can control the symptoms and offer the patient a trouble free period.

Others measures like Yoga, Acupuncture, Meditation and Relaxation techniques are employed to help the patient cope with stressful triggers. The patient is taught to identify his emotions and feelings and learn coping skills to prevent developing mania or depression.

Changing the individual's lifestyle is important like avoiding smoking, alcohol, illicit drugs etc. Certain foods and beverages should be avoided in patients with the disorder. They are caffeine, alcohol, excess sugar, salt, saturated and trans fats. Fast foods and fried items should be reduced. Recommended foods are fruits, vegetables, nuts, salads, and lean meat.

Electroconvulsive Therapy (ECT). *Electroconvulsive Therapy* is helpful in many patients with depressive symptoms and those who are at a risk of suicide. About 80% of patients benefit from ECT. ECT is especially helpful when medications fail to control symptoms.

SCHIZOPHRENIA

Schizophrenia is a mental illness where the person feels detached from the world and has disorganized thinking, hallucinations and delusions. Often the schizophrenia would have started in adult life and is continued into old age. The disease affects all walks of life like family, social life, education, and profession. Often the diagnosis may overlap with symptoms of depression. It is said to affect 1 in 300 people globally.

What are the symptoms of Schizophrenia.

The common symptoms of Schizophrenia are:

1. <u>Delusions</u>. The person often feels strongly about something which is not true or does not exist. He may feel that his thoughts and actions are controlled by someone else outside him.

2. <u>Hallucinations</u>. The person may feel, smell, hear or see things which are not there. E.g., he may smell roses when they are absent. He may hear voices in his ear which compel him to do something. He may see people or objects which are not present. He may hear voices and feel that God is speaking to him.

3. <u>Thinking and Speech</u> . Irrelevant speech and disorganized thinking are hallmarks of the disorder. The patient may feel that others are 'reading' his mind and his thoughts are being 'broadcast' to others. Or he feels that others are 'inserting' thoughts into his mind.

4. <u>Agitation</u>. The person may exhibit severe agitation, irritable, abnormal, and purposeless behavior.

5. He may assume bizarre postures for prolonged periods of time. This is called *Catatonia*.

6. <u>Negative symptoms</u>. The person may be socially withdrawn,

exhibit lack of interest in anything around him, be totally mute, with an expressionless face and unable to feel joy or sorrow.

7. <u>Lack of Self-Care</u>. The person does not take care of himself properly. He does not shave, does not bathe, or comb his hair. He does not care about his clothes.

How is Schizophrenia treated.

The treatment of schizophrenia is done by the Psychiatrist.

<u>Medications</u> are the mainstay of treatment. They are powerful anti-psychotic drugs which have significant side effects and the family members should be made aware of these. In some situations when the patient is violent or has severe symptoms, institutionalization may be needed.

<u>Psychosocial approaches</u> to treatment aim to improve the family life, social life, involvement of family, improving social skills, and job skills. Training in community living and behavioral training are given.

<u>Treatment of co-morbidities</u> like Diabetes, Heart disease, and High blood pressure should be concomitantly followed to prevent complications of these illnesses. Often the patients may not be able to take their medications by themselves and should be helped.

<u>Nutritious food</u>, regular exercise preferably outdoors are encouraged. Group therapy sessions are useful.

SUBSTANCE ABUSE IN THE ELDERLY

Statistics indicates that substance abuse in the elderly in increasing. The overall prevalence is about 4%. The commonly abused substances are Alcohol, prescription medications like Opioids, Benzodiazepines and over the counter preparations. The abuse of substances in the elderly is important as these substances have exaggerated effects in the elderly. The chances of dizziness, falls and unconsciousness after consumption are high leading to fractures, accidents, and head injuries. Not uncommonly, death may occur.

The reason for the substance abuse is varied. Recurrent pain, social isolation, multiple medications for various illnesses, physical disability and poor health are the common causes. Stress due to retirement, financial reasons, family quarrels, bereavement, or problems with sleep may be causative.

Alcohol is the most commonly abused substance and its addiction is not uncommon in the elderly. As the elderly metabolize alcohol at a slower rate, the effects of alcohol are varied in them. High risk drinking where the person drinks more than the permitted number of drinks per day (2 drinks for men and 1 drink for women of hard liquor per day) is seen in two-thirds of elderly over the age of 65. About 10% of the elderly resort to binge drinking which is consuming five or more drinks on one single occasion. Alcohol may cause additional detrimental effects if taken with other prescription medications. Elderly individuals who have diseases of the liver, pancreas or stomach are at a high risk of complications if they consume alcohol.

In 2017, the Centers for Disease Control and Prevention (CDC) reported that about 8% of the elderly above 65 years of age smoked cigarettes. This is important as the risk of heart and lung disease in high in this age group.

Opioid medications for pain are prescribed by physicians for patients with chronic pain and sedatives are prescribed for insomnia. These two classes of drugs are likely to be abused by the elderly.

The elderly person abusing drugs must be treated with a combination of medications and counseling by appropriate qualified practitioners.

Resources.

1. Davidson's Principles and Practice of Medicine. 23rd Edition. 2018 Elsevier. Chapter 28. *Medical Psychiatry*. Pages 1179-1208
2. Depression in Older People. Casarella J . 2022 *Web MD*

https://www.webmd.com/depression/guide/depression-elderly

1. Clinical Practice Guidelines for Geriatric Anxiety Disorders. Subramanyam AA et al. *Indian J Psychiatry*. 2018. 60 : pages 371-382.

https://www.ncbi.nlm.nih.gov/pmc/articles/PMC58409z11/

1. Evaluation and Treatment of Old Age Bipolar Disorder. A Narrative Review. Thampi RR et al. *Drugs in Context*. 2021, 10: pages 1-8.

https://www.ncbi.nlm.nih.gov/pmc/articles/PMC8166731/

1. Schizophrenia in Late Life. Emerging Issues. Folsom DP et al, *Dialogues in Clinical Neuroscience*. 2006, 8 : pages 45-52.

https://www.ncbi.nlm.nih.gov/pmc/articles/PMC3181756/

1. Substance Abuse in Older Adults. Nazario B. 2020. *WebMD*.

https://www.webmd.com/healthy-aging/ss/foods-age-you

8. SEXUALITY IN THE ELDERLY

Sexuality denotes a person's capacity for sexual feelings. It includes the sexual orientation of the person, gender identity, intimacy, eroticism, and social aspects of sex. It includes the sexual feelings of an individual, thoughts, attraction, and behavior towards other people. It is actually the way how we express and experience ourselves sexually. *Intimacy* on the other hand means a feeling of closeness and attachment to the partner. *Ageism* on the other hand means *"the stereotypes (how we think), prejudice (how we feel) and discrimination (how we act) towards others or oneself based on age.* (W.H.O.). It is also used to refer to old people as debilitated, not worthy of employment or attention.

In the United Kingdom it is estimated that by the year 2033, 23% of the population will be above the age of 65. In the United States in 2019, people above the age of 65 represented 16% of the population and were 54.1 million in number. This is expected to rise to 21.6% by 2040.

Many changes occur in people in old age. The changes in the person's body which occurs with aging affects the sexuality of the elderly males and females. There is a decrease in the male and female sex hormones as one ages. There is an atrophy and decrease in size of the reproductive organs along with decrease in function of these organs.

A general deterioration of physical health in both sexes occurs after the age of 65 which may be superimposed with psychological factors like depression and anxiety.

Males have a decrease in the size of the testes and may develop *Erectile Dysfunction.* Both the desire and performance of sex are reduced.

Females have anatomical changes in the vagina and their ovaries. Pain and discomfort during sexual intercourse is felt by them due to the dryness of the vagina and the thinning of the inner lining of the vagina.

To add to this, there are some myths that are perpetuated regarding sexuality in old age. It is falsely believed that nothing can be done for the changes in sexuality that occur in old age, and this must be accepted and endured. The false belief that sex is for the young only and one should give up sex as one grows older is another myth. Other myths ingrained in the mind of many are that sex can lead to a heart attack if you are old and that sexually transmitted diseases do not occur in old age. All this goes to prove that human sexuality is a totally misunderstood topic especially in the elderly.

The problem of sexuality in old age has been studied extensively by psychologists and physicians and multiple research articles are available on this topic.

The elderly individual often hesitates to discuss these problems with his / her medical practitioner due to various reasons. Many elders may come to the doctor along with their adult children and would not be able to voice their concerns in front of them. Others may prefer to discuss their sexual problems only with doctors of the same gender. Social taboos and the culture in which the person was brought up also causes a hesitation in their minds to talk freely about sexuality.

What prevents the elderly from having a normal sex life.

There are multiple factors that prevent the elderly population from having a normal sexual life. One study from Mumbai showed that 72% of individuals below the age of 60 were sexually active whereas only 57% above 60 years were. Some of the reasons for this are discussed below.

- Some elders feel guilty in having sex in old age. This is due to many social taboos and culture in some societies like in India.
- Depression is an important factor in decreasing the sexual drive in the elderly.
- Deteriorating general health and stamina along with any of the illnesses that affect old age like high blood pressure, diabetes, kidney diseases, lung disease, dementia, arthritis, and

surgery for any disease, can lead to a decrease in the sexual drive and loss of interest.

- Stress and anxiety in old age are often causative.
- Medications taken for various illnesses are an important cause of decreasing libido in both males and females. Medications used for high blood pressure, heart diseases, depression, insomnia, and anti-allergic medications can lead to decreased sexual drive.
- *Erectile Dysfunction* (ED) which means difficulty or inability of the male to maintain an erection to have a satisfactory sexual activity may occur due to various diseases like diabetes and neurological illnesses. It may be psychological in some persons.
- The decrease in sex hormones in males and females occurring with aging causes the decrease in sexual drive. In men the decrease in Testosterone causes a delay in sexual arousal and orgasm. In women the decrease in Estrogen causes thinning of vaginal wall, decrease in lubrication and dryness of the vagina leading to pain and discomfort during the sexual act.
- Men may experience changes in ejaculation. It may be premature or delayed in some elders. The quantity of semen produced is decreased.
- The general lack of physical activity and exercise in old age contributes to the decrease in sexuality.
- Women may experience pain during sexual intercourse. Rarely bleeding may occur during intercourse due to the thin vaginal lining being torn.
- Loss of the sexual partner is an important cause for decrease in the sexual urge.
- Many elders fail to find sexual arousal in a new relationship after loss of their regular partner as they might have abstained from sex for a period following the separation. This is called

'Widower's Syndrome'.

Thus, physical changes (what one does) and emotional changes (what one feels) can be the cause of decrease in sexuality in old age.

What can be done to overcome this decrease in sexuality.

The elderly must understand that sexuality in old age is different from that at a younger age, but still is an enjoyable aspect of life. Sex is not only a physically satisfying emotion but is needed for a close emotional connection with the partner. To this end, the elderly must strive to make their sex life satisfying and joyful. In all cases, the root cause of the problem with sexuality must be looked into.

Talking and sharing thoughts with the partner should be part of the elder person's routine. Open communication breeds intimacy which is needed for evoking thoughts of sexuality. Talking about one's problems and feelings is also important to overcome any inhibitions and fears and reintroduce romance in one's life.

Intimate gestures like hugging, touching, and kissing are important in keeping one's spirit alive.

The elderly should make it a point to travel together and have outings and vacations where the intimacy grows.

The lifestyle should be healthy. The diet should be adequate and balanced. Smoking and alc0hol should be excluded. Adequate exercise for both the partners is essential to keep up the physical health. Walking together daily helps develop intimacy, in addition to the exercise it provides. Enough sleep should be ensured.

Stress and anxiety reduction are important part of the management. To this end, there are many methods like relaxation techniques, yoga, meditation, group meetings in clubs etc.

The elderly should approach their primary care physician if they have genuine problems with sexuality. Occasionally hormone replacement may be needed for women. Dryness of the vagina and itching may be relieved by using lubricants or estrogen creams which may be prescribed by the doctor. Men may require testosterone replacement on the advice of the physician.

Any medical causes for the decrease in sexuality should be properly addressed. High blood pressure and diabetes should be kept under control. Other illnesses interfering with the sexual life of the individual should be adequately investigated and treated. Any medications which are the cause for decrease in sexuality in the male or female should be changed.

Erectile dysfunction in the male partner can often be corrected by medications like Sildenafil or Tadalafil which are obtained on the prescription of the medical practitioner. *These drugs should be taken cautiously and are contraindicated in patients with heart disease who are on nitroglycerin or other nitrates for heart disease.*

When necessary, the help of a qualified sex therapist may be sought. Psychotherapy will benefit those who have psychological inhibitions.

At this juncture it is important to caution the readers that one should not be swept away by the false claims of quacks and pharma advertisements regarding 'cures' for waning sexuality in old age. One should be wary of falling into the traps of these charlatans while seeking solace for the problem.

Sex after a Heart Attack

Normally, physiological changes occur in the heart and blood vessels during the sexual act. The work of the heart increases during sexual activity and the heart rate and the blood pressure rise. The maximum increase is during the orgasm and they quickly decrease to normal levels within minutes. This is true for men and women. The physical exertion of sexual activity is equivalent to *climbing two flights of stairs or doing aerobic activity like brisk walking for 10 -15 minutes.*

The fears of sexual activity after a heart attack have been overemphasized in society. It has been found that less than 1% of the individuals develop a heart attack during physical sex. Death during sexual activity is extremely rare. Interestingly it was found that 80-90%

of such deaths occurred in men and almost three-fourth of these cases were in men during *extramarital sex*. Indulging in sex after heavy food intake or a heavy alcoholic binge are risk factors for heart attacks or death during sexual intercourse.

When to resume sexual activity after a heart attack.

Resumption of sexual activity after a heart attack should be gradual. In uncomplicated cases of heart attack, it can be resumed after two to three weeks.

Persons who have had a coronary artery bypass surgery need to wait for 2-3 months before resuming sexual activity for wound healing to be complete. After a Coronary Angioplasty, two to three weeks of rest would suffice before resuming normal sex. Persons who have severe cardiac symptoms like chest pain, breathlessness or heart failure should avoid sex till their symptoms are fully under control.

If a person is able to climb two flights of stairs or walk briskly for 10-15 minutes without symptoms like chest pain (angina), breathlessness or severe fatigue, he/she can resume normal sexual activity.

Gradual resumption of sexual activities implies initial intimacy without physical intercourse and later indulging in physical intercourse. One should avoid sex for at least 3 hours after a heavy meal and avoid heavy alcohol intake before sexual activity. If any symptoms as mentioned above are felt, the individual should immediately stop the activity and take a nitroglycerin tablet prescribed by his medical practitioner.

It has to be cautioned that medications for ED like Sildenafil (Viagra) should never be taken by the patient without consulting his doctor.

After a heart attack, the person should endeavor to return to normal active life before resuming sex. Regular physical exercise resumed gradually is very important in physical reconditioning after a heart attack. The Cardiologist may occasionally advise the patient to perform a Treadmill Exercise Test before resuming his exercise regimen.

<u>Sexual problems in Diabetes.</u>

Diabetic patients may face various sexual issues due to their disease. Long standing diabetes affects the nerves often leading to sexual disorders especially in the males.

Both age and diabetes causes dryness of the vagina in women. This may cause problems like discomfort and pain during sex. Women may have infections of the vagina and some may have urinary incontinence.

The delay in erection and achieving orgasm are the main concerns in men. Failure to maintain erection till ejaculation is another common problem in diabetic men. This is due to the damage to the nerves, muscles and blood vessels supplying the genitals. Rarely a condition called 'Retrograde Ejaculation' occurs where the semen is ejected into the bladder during ejaculation. This, of course, would not be much of a concern in the elderly.

Controlling the blood sugar strictly in both sexes is the most important aspect of treatment. Women need lubricants and estrogen creams or supplements as discussed earlier. Any vaginal infection should be promptly treated.

Men may be given medications for ED by their medical practitioners. Some may need penile devices to overcome the ED. These can be prescribed by their practitioners. The doctor may advise testosterone supplementation as injections if the blood levels of the hormones are low.

Resources

1. Myths about Sexuality and Aging – *Healthy Aging.* 2022

https://blog.kao.kendal.org/myths-about-sexuality-aging?gclid=EAIaIQobChMI8pj7uJy_-wIViClMCh3MmwQMEAAYASAAEgKi3vD_BwE

1. Sexual Activity, Desire, Activity, and Intimacy in the Elderly. Kalra G et al. *Indian J. Psychiatry.* 2011 Oct-Dec; 53(4): 300–306.

https://www.ncbi.nlm.nih.gov/pmc/articles/PMC3267340/

1. Sexual Health. Senior Sex. Tips for Older Men. *Mayo Clinic.* 2022

https://www.mayoclinic.org/healthy-lifestyle/sexual-health/in-depth/senior-sex/art-20046465

1. Women's Sexual Health. Talking About Your Sexual Needs. *Mayo Clinic* 2022

https://www.mayoclinic.org/healthy-lifestyle/sexual-health/in-depth/womens-sexual-health/art-20047771

1. Sexuality in Older Adults. Clinical and Psychosocial Dilemmas. Dhingra I et al. *J. of Geriatric Mental Health.* 2016. 3 : pages. 131-139

https://www.jgmh.org/article.asp?issn=2348-9995;year=2016;volume=3;issue=2;spage=131;epage=139

1. Sexuality and Intimacy in Older Adults. *National Institute of Aging*

https://www.nia.nih.gov/health/sexuality-and-intimacy-older-adults

1. Sexuality in Older Age. Essential Considerations for Healthcare Professionals. Taylor A, Gosney MA. *Age and Ageing.* 2011, 40 : pages 538-543

https://academic.oup.com/ageing/article/40/5/538/46578

1. Sex and Diabetes. American Diabetes Association. 2022.

https://diabetes.org/healthy-living/sexual-health/sex-diabetes

1. Sexual Activity and Cardiovascular Disease. Levine GN et al. *Circulation.* 2012; 125: pages 1058–1072.

https://www.ahajournals.org/doi/full/10.1161/cir.0b013e3182447787

9. SLEEP DISORDERS

Sleep is defined as *"a state of absent wakefulness along with loss of consciousness of one's surroundings when sensory and muscular activity are suspended"*. [6]. It is a resting state when the body is inactive and the mind is unconscious.

Normal Sleep

Sleep is a physiological phenomenon in all animals and man. It is regulated by the Hypothalamus in the brain. The hypothalamus controls the normal 'Sleep-Wake Cycle' or the '*Circadian Rhythm*'. *It is the natural cycle of physical, mental, and behavioral activity of an individual during the 24-hour period.* The hypothalamus in the brain induces the Pineal Gland behind it to secrete a chemical **Melatonin** which induces sleep in the individual. Melatonin produced by the pineal gland is low during day and increases as it becomes dark in the evening. The peak production of melatonin is around 3 am. An elderly person needs sleep for 6-8 hours normally. Lack of sleep is called *Insomnia*.

INSOMNIA

As a person ages, many alterations occur in one's sleep pattern. Elderly people tend to sleep light. They are easily aroused from sleep. Day time sleep increases as one grows old but the total hours spent in sleep decreases. The sleep is interrupted by frequent waking at night – 'fragmented sleep pattern'. The elderly often tend to awaken early. Many of the co-existing diseases like heart disease, neurological diseases and endocrine diseases may affect normal sleep. Medications taken by the elderly for various diseases can affect sleep. It is estimated that about half of the elderly individuals have sleep associated disorders. One group of Psychiatrists found that sleep disorders affected 45% of the elderly in their study group.

What are the causes of Sleep Disorders.

Loss of adequate sleep in the elderly may be due to many causes and consequently lead to problems during daytime.

- Environmental causes like noise, bright light, and extremes of temperature (too cold or too hot) can lead to difficulty in sleeping. Excess humidity in the atmosphere can affect one's sleep. An uncomfortable bed is a common cause.

- The pre-sleep behaviour of the individual can result in problems with sleep. Watching electronic gadgets like smart phones, I-pads, and TV late into the night can lead to problems falling asleep. Lack of exercise during day time is an important cause of lack of sleep. Sleeping during daytime leads to a disturbed sleep at night.

- Medical illnesses in the elderly like heart disease, neurological diseases, allergies, blocked nose, asthma, thyroid problems, and urinary problems can lead to sleep disturbance. Getting up frequently to pass urine as in diabetes, prostate enlargement or urinary infection may disturb sleep. Chronic pain due to any cause may disturb sleep.

- Medications taken by the patient for high blood pressure, asthma, and other diseases, steroids and anti-depressants, may lead to sleep disorders.
- Stress and Anxiety in the elderly is an important cause of insomnia.
- Alcohol, Caffeine, and smoking can lead to difficulty in sleeping.
- Travel between time zones can cause Jet Lag in individuals. The elderly are more prone to the adverse effects of jet lag compared to the young.
- Other causes like death of a spouse, loneliness and hospitalization affect sleep.
- In addition, there are primary sleep disorders of which Restless Leg Syndrome and Sleep Apnea are important and will be dealt with later in this chapter.

What are the effects of Sleep Deprivation.

Improper sleep at night may lead to many daytime problems in the elderly individuals.

- Feeling fatigued and lethargic during daytime is a consequence of inadequate or disturbed sleep at night. They feel an overall reduction in stamina.
- The attention span of the individual and the ability to concentrate are affected.
- Daytime sleepiness may occur and can be dangerous in some individuals leading to accidents while driving, mishaps in the kitchen or while using appliances or machinery.
- Mood changes may occur in the persons who are sleep deprived and they may become irritable, aggressive, or easily annoyed.

- Sleep deprivation can lead to poor performance in professional and social interactions.

How can lack of sleep be managed.

Changes need to be made in lifestyle of the elderly person. Medications are needed only when the lifestyle changes fail to improve their sleep pattern.

Lifestyle Changes. Having a regular 'Sleep Hygiene' is important in getting to sleep. In the majority of individuals this change in lifestyle can lead to a better sleep pattern. Some of the suggestions are as follows.

- Regular aerobic physical exercise is necessary for the elderly to have a proper lifestyle conducive to a healthy sleep hygiene. Exercises should be done in the early morning or evening. Exercise just before going to bed must be avoided.
- Stimulants like caffeine, cocoa, alcohol, or smoking should be avoided before bedtime.
- The sleeping environment of the person should be quiet and dark. Lights should be switched off, though a night lamp may be permitted in the elderly. The bed room should be free of noise. Loud music should be avoided, but soft soothing music may be helpful for some persons. Essential oils derived from plants like lavender, chamomile, eucalyptus, cedar wood and sandalwood have been found to induce a pleasant sleep. Such aromatherapy is regularly used by some in their bed rooms. These oils may be applied to the skin, used in a diffuser or humidifier, or put on one's pillow to provide a soothing fragrance at night.
- The room temperature should be maintained at 75°F or 24°C for comfort. Air conditioning is ideal.
- Meals should be taken at regular times of the day. Snacks if needed, may be taken, but heavy meals before bedtime should

be avoided. The evening meal (dinner) should be taken sufficiently early, say by 6 – 6.30 pm so that digestion is partly over by the time the person retires to bed. A light snack may be permitted at bed time if the person feels hungry.

- Fluid intake should be limited prior to bedtime to avoid getting up frequently to pass urine. Coffee should be avoided for at least 4-5 hours before going to bed.

- The person should be encouraged to go to bed only when feeling sleepy and the bed used only for sleeping. Working in bed, watching TV, or indulging in social media chats while in bed are to be discouraged. *Blue light exposure from electronic gadgets prior to sleep should be avoided as it blocks the release of melatonin from the brain.*

- The elderly should accustom themselves to get up at the same time daily morning and go to bed at the same time at night. This establishes a routine of a proper sleep-wake cycle in them.

- During daytime, they should expose themselves to bright daylight as much as possible by exercising outdoors whenever possible.

- Having a glass of warm milk (or some cheese) before going to bed ensures a good sleep in some persons. It is found that two compounds namely, Tryptophan and Melatonin in milk promote sleep. Interestingly, it has been found that the milk from cows milked at night contains more of Melatonin.

- For those who still have problems with sleep, relaxation techniques like breathing exercises (*Pranayama*), meditation and muscle relaxation techniques are helpful.

Medications for Sleep. These are available but should be avoided as far as possible if the lifestyle changes work for an individual. Some medications like Melatonin, Diphenhydramine, or Doxylamine are available over the counter. These should be used in the smallest dose needed and only for short periods. Prolonged use may cause habituation. These drugs may produce side effects like fatigue and day time drowsiness and should be used with caution.

Stronger medications for sleep disorders are available on prescription from the doctor and should be used only on medical advice and for short periods at a time.

RESTLESS LEG SYNDROME (RLS)

This is a condition characterized by disturbing sensations in the legs associated with an overwhelming urge to move the legs. It is seen more during periods of rest like sitting or lying down to sleep and hence may cause disturbances of sleep. It is seen in about 7 – 10% of adults. RLS may be a significant cause of sleep disturbance in the elderly population.

What are the symptoms of RLS.

The disturbance is seen more towards the evening and night in most of the affected individuals and is increased when the person is resting. Periods of prolonged rest as occurs during flights, traveling in a car or watching a movie at night induce the symptoms.

The person feels a sensation of itching, crawling, tickling, aching or creeping sensation in the legs and feels compelled to move the legs to prevent this abnormal sensation. The symptoms decrease when he gets up and walks. He may feel relieved when he constantly moves his legs. While in bed the person constantly moves his legs or tosses in bed from side to side. These movements are often involuntary and the person may not be aware of them.

During daytime, the person does not feel the symptoms. Such episodes of restlessness of the legs may last for days together and at times disappear only to reappear after some time.

Rarely, these abnormal sensations and compulsion to move the limbs may occur in the arms.

Diseases like kidney diseases, neurological diseases, iron deficiency, using medications for vomiting, alcohol, nicotine, and caffeine may also produce similar symptoms of RLS. Diabetic neuropathy where the disease involves the peripheral nerves may cause RLS.

The cause for this disorder is unknown but it is seen in first degree relatives of the patient and hence is thought to have a genetic basis.

How is RLS treated.

Many methods of treatment have been used in the condition.

- If any specific cause like kidney disease, iron deficiency or diabetic neuropathy is detected, they are treated appropriately.
- The patient is advised to follow a regular pattern of sleep, going to bed, and waking up at fixed times daily.
- Regular exercise during daytime may relieve the night time symptoms to a great extent. Stretching exercises especially to the legs are advocated. Yoga is a good example of stretching exercise.
- A warm bath in the evening benefits some patients.
- Avoidance of alcohol and tobacco is important.
- Massage to the legs is beneficial in some. The habit of having a massage to the legs using medicated oil (*Ayurvedic*) followed by a warm bath is usually the custom in countries like India where many elderly individuals follow this practice.
- Some patients derive benefit from using heating pads in the legs or a warm electric blanket at night during sleep.
- Medications are available for the treatment of RLS and are mainly those used for seizures (epilepsy). Sedative medications provide benefit to some patients. Occasionally opioid medications may be needed.

The disease is often lifelong with periods of remission and exacerbation and many patients learn to adjust their lifestyle as there is no permanent cure.

SLEEP APNEA SYNDROME (SAS)

Sleep Apnea Syndrome also called **Obstructive Sleep Apnea (OSA)** is seen in about 13-32% of the elderly population and causes significant disturbances of sleep.

It is caused mainly by a decrease in the tone of the muscles of the throat leading to narrowing of the airways in the throat during sleep resulting in a decrease in breathing. In addition, the tongue may fall back in some patients during sleep increasing the narrowing of the upper airway.

What causes OSA.

When a normal person sleeps, breathing – movement of air into and out of the lungs - decreases by 10-15%. When the person is awake, there is a voluntary increase in breathing in all individuals. the narrowing of the airway in the throat which occurs in patients with OSA causes a further decrease in breathing leading to a lowering of oxygen contained in the blood. The patient continues to breathe and may have transient periods when he stops breathing. This short period of absent breathing is called *Apnea*. Within seconds, the person resumes breathing normally. These cycles of normal breathing interspersed with short periods of apnea are the characteristic feature of OSA.

Males are more prone to develop OSA. So are smokers and those with a family history of OSA.

Narrowing of the throat and upper airway may occur due to enlargement of the tonsils or due to the presence of a narrow airway in some people even from childhood.

Obese persons with thick necks are at a significant risk of developing this disorder. It may be seen in diseases like heart failure, diabetes, chronic kidney disease and certain lung diseases.

Use of alcohol and sedatives is associated with OSA. Some patients with chronic nasal congestion due to diseases like allergy or sinusitis are prone to develop OSA.

What are the symptoms of OSA.

The cyclical breathing punctuated by periods of transient apnea are the classical feature of OSA. During the short period when they stop breathing, they may awaken with a loud gasp or cough.

Patients with OSA often snore loudly during sleep. _But all persons who snore do not have OSA_. Sleep is often disturbed by this frequent awakening.

Patients with OSA often have daytime drowsiness and lethargy. They may have mild cognitive dysfunction and inability to concentrate or perform skillful actions.

They may develop headache during the day. The blood pressure is often found to be high in patients with OSA.

What complications can OSA lead to.

OSA can cause some complications in individuals, especially the elderly.

- It has been found that these patients have drowsiness during daytime which can pose a potential hazard to themselves and others during driving and handling machinery. They are accident prone. They may have mood swings, may be irritable and easily annoyed.
- Cardiovascular problems like high blood pressure, heart failure, stroke, heart attacks and irregularities of the heart (Arrhythmias) are more common in patients with OSA.
- They are highly sensitive to medications like sedatives and those given for anesthesia.
- Increased chances of post operative complications following any surgery is seen in these patients.
- Increase in pressure inside the eyeball causing a condition called Glaucoma is seen in patients with OSA. (See section on

The Eye)

- Males with OSA may have problems with sexual function and erectile dysfunction.

How is OSA diagnosed.

Diagnosis of this condition is by observing the patient in a laboratory while sleeping. Tests are performed to detect the changes during sleep. This is called *Polysomnography* or 'Sleep Study'. The patient is tested in a Sleep Laboratory where he is connected to a variety of monitors during sleep and his heart, breathing pattern, blood oxygen levels and brain function are monitored. This gives the physician an accurate idea of the problem so as to plan appropriate treatment.

Others tests to diagnose any co-existing conditions like heart disease, kidney disease or lung disease may also be done.

How is OSA treated.

Some of the methods of treatment are:

- Lifestyle modification is needed to achieve an ideal body weight. Obesity should be treated.
- Regular aerobic exercise is advised.
- Alcohol in excess and smoking should be avoided.
- Sedative medications and anti-anxiety medications are best avoided as they can aggravate the OSA.
- The patient is encouraged to sleep to one side and avoid sleeping on his back. This can be aided by stitching a tennis ball to the back of the patient's T-shirt or clothing so that he does not involuntarily lie on his back during sleep. Packing pillows on either side can also help him lie on his side.
- Any underlying condition in the patient leading to OSA should be treated. E.g., Tonsil enlargement, Sinusitis, Heart failure.
- If nasal congestion is present, a nasal spray at bedtime should

be helpful.

- A specialized device using a face mask is used to apply pressure to the upper airway when the patient is asleep. This is called **Positive Airway breathing**. It is a bit cumbersome and all patients may not tolerate it. Applying high pressure to the airway prevents it from narrowing while breathing and relieves the OSA.

- Surgical methods to correct any narrowing of the upper airway like surgical removal of tonsils, correction of nasal passage obstruction or jaw surgery are done in some patients to correct OSA.

JET LAG

Modern aeronautic technology and travel has shortened distances so that people travel between time zones very often. One casualty of this travel across several time zones is the disturbance in sleep rhythm. This is called *Jet Lag*. Our body's circadian rhythm is normally synchronized with the original time zone where we dwell. When we move to a new time zone, our body takes some time to adjust to the new time zone and hence our sleep-wake cycle is temporarily disrupted.

Jet lag is experienced when a person crosses more than *three time zones* when traveling. Some people travel across multiple time zones within a short span of time like traveling to India from the United States on a jet liner. The time zones between these two countries is 10 ½ hours or more and hence many time zones are crossed.

What are the symptoms of Jet Lag.

Symptoms of jet lag varies from person to person. The elderly experience more jet lag symptoms unlike the young who get adjusted easily. Some people develop multiple symptoms whereas others have only one symptom -usually a sleep disorder.

- The commonest symptom of Jet lag is disordered sleep. It is seen either as an inability to fall asleep or early awakening. This depends on whether the person has traveled east or west from where he was living. It takes a few days to overcome this till the body adjusts to the new surroundings and time zone.
- Fatigue and lethargy during daytime and a dazed feeling are common.
- The person is unable to concentrate or focus on a problem or work. Mood changes like irritability may be seen in some persons.
- Some individuals develop diarrhea or constipation along with indigestion.

- Headaches are not uncommon.

What causes Jet Lag.

The main cause of Jet Lag is an asynchronous circadian rhythm till the body adjusts to the new time zone.

The low cabin pressure in the aircraft adds to the development of this disorder.

The low humidity in the aircraft tends to cause dehydration and this further adds to the symptoms of Jet Lag.

Flying eastward tends to cause more Jet lag than flying westward.

The more time zones one crosses, the severe are the symptoms and they persist for more number of days. Roughly it is said that it takes one day per time zone crossed for full recovery to occur.

The elderly are often more jet lagged than the younger persons.

The main danger of jet lag is accidents. Accidents may occur while driving and while manipulating machinery. Errors in decision making may occur when a person is severely jet lagged.

How can Jet Lag be treated.

Often this does not need any treatment. Preventive measures detailed below are helpful in avoiding it to a large extent.

Sunlight is the best remedy for jet lag. After traveling to a new time zone, the person should endeavor to expose himself to sunlight during the day time in the new time zone. Bright light falling on the retina of the eye causes signals to reach the hypothalamus which in turn suppresses the release of melatonin from the pineal gland. If one has traveled *East*, sunlight exposure in the *mid-morning and noon* is helpful and if traveled towards the *West, late afternoon* exposure helps.

Light therapy has been used as a method of overcoming jet lag. The person is exposed for some time to artificial bright light similar to sunlight so that daytime is simulated and the brain is tricked into believing that it is morning.

Daytime sleepiness may be overcome by drinking coffee to keep awake and alert. Adequate exercise during day time is also helpful.

Medications like sedatives may be used. Melatonin is available as tablets which may be taken 30 minutes before going to bed in a small dose of 1-3 mg.

How can we prevent Jet Lag.

Some preventive measures may be taken well before traveling to avoid or mitigate the effects of jet lag.

- One should take adequate rest before traveling. Hectic activities are better avoided on the day of travel.
- If one plans to travel towards the east, beginning a few days prior to travel, one should go to bed 1 – 2 hours early so as to adjust to the time zone in the destination. If traveling west, one should go to bed 1-2 hours later than usual for a few days prior to travel.
- Similarly, the person should expose oneself to sunlight *before* traveling. If going *East* expose oneself to *morning sunlight* and if going *West*, to *evening sunlight* for a few days prior to the travel date.
- During the flight, one should take care to drink adequate fluids like juices or water. Avoid alcohol and coffee during the flight if possible.
- One should eat sparingly prior to travel and during the flight. Heavy meals inflight should be avoided.
- If one is reaching the destination at night, maximum amount sleep on the plane should be obtained.
- Once the destination is reached, the person should not sleep during daytime. Meals should be eaten at the local times in the destination. To keep awake, coffee helps.
- If one feels extremely sleepy during day, short naps of 15-20 minutes (not more) may be taken.

Resources

1. Davidson's Principles and Practice of Medicine 23rd edition. Elsevier. 2018. *Disorders of Sleep*. Pages. 1105-1106.
2. Sleep Disorders in the Elderly. Diagnosis & Management. Suzuki K et al. *Journal of General & Family Medicine*. 2017;18:61–71.

https://www.ncbi.nlm.nih.gov/pmc/articles/
PMC5689397/#!po=48.6842

1. Restless Leg Syndrome Fact Sheet. *National Institute of Neurological Disorders & Stroke*. 2022.

https://www.ninds.nih.gov/restless-legs-syndrome-fact-
sheet#:~:text=Restless%20legs%20syndrome%20(RLS)%2C,sitting%20or%20ly[1].

1. Sleep Apnea in Older People. Glasser M et al. *Breathe*. 2011 7: Pages 248-256.

https://breathe.ersjournals.com/content/7/3/
248#:~:text=Summary%20Obstructive%20sleep%20apnoea%20is,the%20defini[2].

---

1. https://www.ninds.nih.gov/restless-legs-syndrome-fact-
sheet#_853ae90f0351324bd73ea615e6487517__4c761f170e016836ff84498202b99827__853ae90f0351324bd73ea615e6487517_text_43ec3e5dee6e706af7766fffea512721_Restless_0bcef9c45bd8a48eda1b26eb0c61c869_20legs_0bcef9c45bd8a48eda1b26eb0c61c869_20syndrome_0bcef9c45bd8a48eda1b26eb0c61c869_20_84c40473414caf2ed4a7b1283e48bbf4_RLS_9371d7a2e3ae86a00aab4771e39d255d__0bcef9c45bd8a48eda1b26eb0c61c869_2C_c0cb5f0fcf239ab3d9c1fcd31fff1efc_sitting_0bcef9c45bd8a48eda1b26eb0c61c869_20or_0bcef9c45bd8a48eda1b26eb0c61c869_20lying_0bcef9c45bd8a48eda1b26eb0c61c869_20in_0bcef9c45bd8a48eda1b26eb0c61c869_20bed

2. https://breathe.ersjournals.com/content/7/3/
248#_853ae90f0351324bd73ea615e6487517__4c761f170e016836ff84498202b99827__853ae90f0351324bd73ea615e6487517_text_43ec3e5dee6e706af7766fffea512721_Summary_0bcef9c45bd8a48eda1b26eb0c61c869_20Obstructive_0bcef9c45bd8a48eda1b26eb0c61c869_20sleep_0bcef9c45bd8a48eda1b26eb0c61c869_20apnoea_0bcef9c45bd8a48eda1b26eb0c61c869_20is_c0cb5f0fcf239ab3d9c1fcd31fff1efc_the_0bcef9c45bd8a48eda1b26eb0c61c869_20definitions_0bcef9c45bd8a48eda1b26eb0c61c869_20of_0bcef9c45bd8a48eda1b26eb0c61c869_20the_0bcef9c45bd8a48eda1b26eb0c61c869_20disease

1. Jet Lag. Atkinson G et al. *Traveler's Health*. Chapter 8 Travel by Air, Land and Sea. 2020.

https://wwwnc.cdc.gov/travel/yellowbook/2020/travel-by-air-land-sea/jet-lag

1. Buysse DJ. Sleep Health. Can we define it ? Does it matter ? *Sleep* 37 : pages 9-17, 2014.

10. TEMPERATURE REGULATION

Man is warm blooded. It means that the human body maintains a constant temperature which is different from the normal atmospheric temperature. The body temperature is perfectly maintained within a narrow normal range. The normal body temperature is 37° Celsius or 98.6° Fahrenheit. The body maintains its temperature in a close range between 35 and 39 degree Celsius.

How does the normal body regulate the Temperature.

The maintenance of normal temperature is called *Thermoregulation*. The human body efficiently regulates body heat by various mechanisms as the body's metabolic functions take place optimally within the narrow range of temperature.

The Hypothalamus in the brain (See section on *Brain* in Book1) is the Thermoregulatory center in the brain. It functions like a thermostat and detects any change in body temperature and takes immediate action to set the temperature back to normal. When the ambient temperature is hot, the body tends to lose heat and when the temperature outside is cold, the body tends to conserve heat.

The **Core Body Temperature** denotes the temperature of the internal organs of the body like the liver, heart, blood, brain etc. It is normally maintained within a narrow range of 36.5°C and 37.4 °C.

When the body temperature tends to rise due to increase in the temperature outside, the blood vessels of the skin dilate. More blood flows into the skin and the heat from the blood is dissipated to the outside atmosphere. This heat loss from the skin is more in the hands, feet, ears, nose tips, cheeks, and ears. Hence the importance of covering these areas in cold weather when we do not want to lose body heat. In addition, in hot weather, the sweat glands in the skin increase the production of sweat and this cools down the skin and the body as the sweat evaporates.

Conversely, when the ambient temperature turns cold, the body mechanisms to conserve heat kick in. the skin blood vessels *constrict* or become very narrow thereby reducing the heat lost from the skin. Sweating stops and thus heat is conserved. A third mechanism to conserve heat is Shivering. Shivering increases the muscle activity which generates heat. This heat is distributed by the blood to the inner core of the body to keep the internal organs normally warm.

What happens to Thermoregulation in the Elderly.

As one ages, changes occur in the body which interfere with normal thermoregulation and this leads to the elderly individual's inability to tolerate extremes of heat or cold like the young.

1. The ability of the skin blood vessels to *dilate* or *constrict* is reduced in old age thereby affecting the temperature control system. Hence, in cold climates, the body is unable to conserve its core temperature and in hot climates, it is not able to lose heat as efficiently as before.

2. The sweat glands in the elderly produce less sweat in response to increased environmental temperatures. Hence heat loss from the body is reduced.

3. Subcutaneous fat is reduced in old age. The subcutaneous fat normally functions as an insulation to conserve heat during cold weather. Loss of fat hence causes the inability to tolerate cold.

4. As body muscle mass is reduced in the elderly, shivering is not able to produce as much heat as it would produce in a young person.

5. The blood flow to the skin normally changes rapidly to conserve or lose heat from the body. This ability to dilate to lose heat and constrict to conserve heat is decreased as one ages.

Causes and Risk Factors leading to Temperature-Related illnesses in the elderly.

There are many causes of intolerance to heat and cold. Some of the important causes are:

1. The ability to tolerate extremes of environmental temperature decreases after the age of 60. But temperature intolerance is most obvious in those above the age of 70 and 80.

2. Fatigue and tiredness due to any cause decreases the tolerance of the individual to changes in external temperature.

3. Many medical conditions can render an individual incapable of adjusting to temperature variations. Hypothyroidism, undernutrition, frailty, stroke, and arthritis may make the patients intolerant to cold. Similarly, Hyperthyroidism makes them unable to tolerate heat.

4. Most of the elderly individuals are on medication for co-existing illnesses. Some of these medications can cause intolerance to temperature. Antidepressants, narcotic medications, sedatives, drugs for high blood pressure and heart diseases may render temperature regulation inadequate.

5. Alcohol, though it gives a false sense of warmth in the person, is really harmful in cold weather. It reduces shivering, increases the blood flow to skin thereby causing heat loss rather than conservation. Alcohol also affects the judgement of the individual leading to wrong decision making.

6. Patients who have mental illness, may not be able to take proper decisions to adjust to the climate change and are at a disadvantage.

7. Bedridden patients as in paralyzed patients and those with stroke or fractures may not be able to adjust to the external temperature changes and are vulnerable to heat or cold related illnesses.

8. Elderly individuals living alone in homes or apartments which

are not climate controlled are also at a high risk of developing such illnesses.

HEAT RELATED ILLNESSES

Older adults are unable to adjust to increase in atmospheric temperature and it may result in serious illnesses in them. It is more pronounced in individuals who have co-existing illnesses like Heart disease, Diabetes, Stroke, Parkinson's disease, or extensive skin disease.

The heat-related illnesses in the elderly are Heat Stroke, Heat Exhaustion, Heat Cramps, Sunburn and Heat Rash.

<u>Heat Stroke</u>.

Heat stroke is the severest form of heat-related illness where the body temperature shoots up to levels of **103°F** or higher. The skin becomes hot and dry and the patient may have nausea, vomiting or severe headache. <u>Sweating is often absent</u> as the thermoregulatory mechanism fails in extreme temperature. Often they are dizzy, confused and may lose consciousness.

The patient should be immediately removed to a cool place and given cold compresses with a towel soaked in cold water. The compresses are given to the neck, groins, armpits, and chest wall. Cold water sponge bath is helpful. Sips of cold water or juice should be given. *Alcohol or caffeinated drinks should never be given.* Immediate hospitalization is needed as this may turn fatal.

In the hospital, the patient is cooled externally and also internally by using equipment which cool the blood which is circulated through them. External cooling is done using ice packs and cooling blankets. Cold *saline* or glucose is infused intravenously.

Untreated, heat stroke can lead to kidney or liver failure, fall of blood pressure, swelling of the brain or fluid collection in the lungs. Fatality is not uncommon if the patient is not treated in time. The earlier the treatment is given, the lesser the chances of complications and death.

<u>Heat Exhaustion</u>

This often accompanies exertion in hot weather as in farm workers and laborers who work outdoors in hot, humid climates. Unlike heat stroke, the patient exhibits <u>severe sweating</u> with a cold clammy skin, severe tiredness, headache, dizziness, nausea and vomiting, muscle cramps, fast heart rate and a fall in blood pressure.

The immediate treatment is to remove the person from the hot environment and cool the individual using the techniques described above. The patients are often dehydrated and fluids should be given orally or intravenously.

Heat Cramps

Heavy exertion and sweating in hot weather can lead to heat cramps. The patient experiences painful muscle contractions occurring in the legs, arms, or abdominal muscles. It is associated with <u>severe sweating</u> and is due to decrease in sodium. The patient's body temperature does not rise.

Treatment consists in removing the person to a cool area and providing cool liquids containing salt to drink. ORS solution, fruit juices or salted *buttermilk* are ideal. Some patients may need intravenous *saline*.

Heat Edema

This is a condition where the feet, legs or hands swell when the external temperatures are high. It is not dangerous and the treatment is to elevate the feet. Salt intake should be *decreased*.

Sunburn

Exposure to sun's ultraviolet rays may cause sunburn on exposed areas of the body. The skin is red, hot, and painful to touch. Occasionally blisters may appear.

If pain is severe, a pain relieving tablet can be taken. The skin should be cooled with cool compresses. A moisturizing cream may be applied. The skin may peel after a couple of days.

Heat Rash (Prickly Heat)

This is due to the openings of the sweat glands (*pores*) in the skin being blocked causing sweat to be trapped in the skin. It causes multiple, tiny swellings and occasionally smally blisters in the skin. These are seen in clusters on the skin. The neck, chest, groin, elbow, and creases of skin are usually involved. It occurs in the covered areas of the body.

Treatment consists of avoiding direct sunlight, having a cool bath, use of cool compresses and dusting with dry talcum powder. Creams and ointments should be avoided as these may further block the openings of the sweat glands.

How to prevent Heat-related Illnesses.

Certain precautions are needed to prevent heat related illnesses.

- One should avoid exposure to the sun's rays between 10 am and 4 pm when the UV rays are the maximum.

- Exercising in hot climates should be avoided.
- When outdoors, elderly individuals should remain in the shade as far as possible,.
- Light cotton clothes of light colors should preferably worn in summer. Clothes made of synthetic fabric should not be worn in hot weather.
- Regular exercises should be done so as to keep one's muscles strong and prevent muscle loss in old age.
- The elderly should be well hydrated and drink plenty of water. They may not feel thirst like the young individuals. Hence, they should remember to drink fluids at frequent intervals even if not thirsty. Alcohol and caffeine containing beverages should be avoided in hot weather.
- Salt and water should be replaced when there is excess sweating. (See section on *Dehydration* in Book1).
- Heavy meals and hot, spicy dishes should be eschewed.
- Staying indoors during the hot days and keeping the shades

and curtains in the home closed during the hot days, is preferable.

- Being in an air-conditioned environment is preferable.
- Cooking using oven or stove is better avoided.
- The elderly should take adequate rest during the day time.
- A cooling shower or immersing one's feet in cold water in a basin are methods to keep one's body cool.
- Wearing sunscreen lotion with a Sun Protection Factor (SPF) of 15 or above, 30 minutes before going outdoors in the sun should be advised.
- Patients with co-morbidities should do their outdoor chores in the mornings or evenings without exposing to the hot sun's rays.
- Children or the elderly should not be left alone in the car in hot weather.
- Elderly individuals living alone should be checked regularly by their relatives or caregivers for any signs of dehydration or symptoms of heat-related illness.

COLD-RELATED ILLNESSES

Even though there are cold-related illnesses like frostbite and chilblains, we shall discuss only Hypothermia in this section.

<u>Hypothermia</u>

The core body temperature tends to fall when the environmental temperature becomes very low. When the core body temperature falls *below 95°F or 35°C*, the metabolic functions of the body slow down which may ultimately lead to death. This condition is called **Hypothermia**. This unusually low body temperature affects the brain causing the patient to become confused and consequently unable to act to get out of the situation. Exposure to cold weather and immersion in cold water can lead to hypothermia.

In the early stages of hypothermia, the patient may have shivering, mental confusion, and dizziness. Later, he may gradually slip into unconsciousness as the condition worsens. The breathing and pulse become slow, the speech becomes slurred and the patient becomes unresponsive. The lips, skin and nails may appear blue due to severe constriction of the skin blood vessels. The presence of diseases like Hypothyroidism, liver or kidney disease, and stroke makes a person more vulnerable to hypothermia. The core body temperature drops and ultimately the heart may stop beating leading to death of the individual.

As soon as hypothermia is detected or suspected, the person should be removed to a warm area. Wet clothes should be removed and the patient covered with layers of blankets. A warm electric blanket may be used.

Warm drinks may be given. *Alcoholic beverages should never be given.* Heat should not be applied directly to the skin.

If the patient has a cardiac arrest, Cardiopulmonary Resuscitation *(CPR)* should be started immediately. In a hospital, treatment consists of external rewarming using warm air, blankets, warm pads, or warm baths. Internal rewarming is done by warming the blood outside using a Heart-Lung machine and infusing it back into the patient. Other methods of rewarming the patient internally to raise the core temperature are also available in the hospitals.

Prevention of Hypothermia and Cold-related illnesses.

Elderly individuals should take adequate precautions to avoid getting cold-related illnesses.

- Those with other co-existing illnesses should avoid cold exposure.

- Children and the elderly should take care to stay warm in cold weather. Woolen, silk, or clothes made of synthetic fabrics may be worn in layers in cold weather especially when going outdoors. The head, neck, ears, hands, and feet should be covered with adequate clothing like scarves, cap, hoods, gloves, and socks. Wind resistant clothing should be worn outdoors.

- Exertion in cold weather should be avoided.

- One should keep dry in cold weather and change any wet clothing immediately.

- Shivering is an early warning sign that one should not ignore. If shivering occurs, one should move to a warm area.

- Consuming alcoholic beverages in cold weather is not advised. It gives a false sense of warmth. Smoking should be avoided.

- When it is snowing, the elderly should remain indoors. They are liable to slip and fall on wet surfaces and snow-covered areas.

- Lip balm should be applied to prevent drying and cracking of lips. Vaseline may suffice. Similarly, the skin should be kept moist by using moisturizing cream immediately after a bath.

- Bathing should be in *warm* water and not in *hot* water.

- Drinking warm water frequently is advised.

- A healthy, nutritious diet with plenty of fruits and vegetables to keep one's energy levels up should be consumed.

- The indoor temperature should be kept at 68 - 70°F by adjusting the thermostat.
- If one is driving alone, the mobile phone and charger should be kept in the car. A blanket and water to drink should always be carried in the car.
- Elders living alone should be checked regularly by their relatives or caregivers.

Refer to the section on Skin regarding dry skin in cold weather.

Resources

1. Davidson's Principles and Practice of Medicine. 23rd Edition. Elsevier. 2018. *Chapter 9-Environmental Medicine* pages 163-172

2. Thermoregulation and Aging. Van Someren EJW. *Amer J. Physiol Regul Integr Comp Physiol* 2007. 292 – R99-R102. PO.

https://journals.physiology.org/doi/full/10.1152/ajpregu.00557.2006

1. Aging and Thermoregulatory Control: The Clinical Implications of Exercising Under Heat Stress in Older Individuals. Balmain BN et al. *Biomed Research International*. 2018, Vol.2018: 8306154.

https://www.ncbi.nlm.nih.gov/pmc/articles/
PMC6098859/#__ffn_sectitle

1. Warning Signs and Symptoms of Heat Related Illness. Natural Disasters and Severe Weather *Centers for Disease Control & Prevention*. 2017

https://www.cdc.gov/disasters/extremeheat/warning.html

1. Accidental Hypothermia in Adults. *UpToDate*. Zafren K. Mechem CC. 2022.

https://www.uptodate.com/contents/accidental-hypothermia-in-adults

11. MISCELLANEOUS CONDITIONS

After having discussed many of the systems in the human body and their ailments in old age, let us briefly look at a few common miscellaneous problems which trouble the elderly. These may be asymptomatic to begin with posing no difficulties or distress to the person. But in some individuals they may be troublesome needing medical attention.

The diseases which are being dealt with here are Benign Prostatic Hypertrophy, Hernia, Hemorrhoids, Cervical Spondylosis, Back pain, and Frailty.

BENIGN PROSTATIC HYPERTROPHY (BPH)

The prostate is a small walnut sized gland that sits below the urinary bladder in front of the rectum in males. The urethra passes through it from the bladder before continuing into the penis. As one grows old the prostate gland enlarges in size due to multiplication of cells within it. This is called Benign Prostatic Hypertrophy (**BPH**) and usually begins after the age of 50. By the age of 60 about half of the males have some signs of BPH. By the age of 85, 90% of males have signs of BPH, but only half of them have symptoms which need treatment.

BPH is due to the decrease in the male hormone, Testosterone as one ages and the relative increase in the female hormone estrogen. Persons with a family history of BPH tend to get the disease. Those suffering from diabetes, and heart disease have a higher chance of developing BPH. (See section on *Kidneys & Urinary System* in Book 1). *It must be remembered that BPH does not necessarily lead to development of Prostate cancer.*

What are the symptoms of BPH.

In many elderly individuals, the enlargement may not be accompanied by any symptoms but is detected on routine physical examination or during an ultrasound scanning of the abdomen. The common symptoms with which a person presents are:

- An increase in the frequency of passing urine is often the commonest symptom. The quantity of urine passed each time may be small. The patient often has to get up many times at night to pass urine. A patient having to pass urine more than twice at night should be suspected of having BPH.
- Difficulty in initiating urination is another common symptom. The patient has to wait for some time before he can initiate passing urine and often feels the need to strain. This

symptom is called **Hesitancy.**

- Occasionally, the patient feels an intense urge to pass urine and unless he reaches the toilet immediately, may soil his undergarments. This symptom is called **Precipitancy.**
- The urine stream may be thin while passing urine.
- A feeling of incomplete emptying of the bladder is present even after passing sufficient quantity of urine.
- After passing urine there may be dribbling of a few drops of urine which continues for some time, often soiling the clothes.
- In some patients there may be symptoms of urinary incontinence. They may inadvertently pass urine while coughing, sneezing, laughing or straining to lift a heavy weight.
- Some patients present with repeated urinary tract infections and may pass blood in urine. The urine may have a bad smell.
- Pain while passing urine or while ejaculating may be felt by some.

What complications may occur in BPH.

If BPH is left untreated despite symptoms, it can lead to complications in the elderly individual.

Backflow of urine from the bladder into the ureters can lead to damage to the ureters and kidneys resulting in chronic kidney failure.

Repeated urinary infections in some patients can cause kidney damage.

Due to the obstruction of the urethra in the prostate gland, urine may accumulate in the bladder leading to stretching of the bladder wall. This may cause the muscles of the bladder to become weak and the bladder enlarges in size and cannot empty properly.

The stagnant urine in the bladder may give rise to stones.

Occasionally, the patient may have a sudden and total inability to pass urine and the bladder enlarges causing acute distress. This is called **Acute Urinary Retention** and should be relieved immediately by passing a catheter into bladder to drain the urine.

How is BPH diagnosed.

The disease is diagnosed based on the history of difficulty in urination given by the patient. In addition, the *Urologist* does a rectal examination of the patient. A gloved finger is introduced through the anus into the patient's rectum and the prostate gland is felt. Its size and enlargement is thus determined by the doctor.

An Ultrasound examination of the abdomen shows the prostate enlargement its size can be measured. The size of the bladder and any residual urine in the bladder can be determined.

An instrument named Cystoscope is passed into the bladder through the urethra and the inside of the bladder inspected by the doctor. This procedure called Cystoscopy gives the doctor more details about the bladder.

Routine tests of blood and urine are also done. A specific test in blood detects a protein named Prostate Specific Antigen (PSA). This may increase in many conditions including BPH, infection in the prostate, after surgery of the prostate and in Prostate cancer. *It is to be noted that increase in PSA does not always mean Prostate Cancer.*

A biopsy of the prostate is done as a part of the investigation to rule out the possibility of cancer of the prostate and to diagnose benign hypertrophy.

How is BPH treated.

Many patients have enlargement of the prostate when they grow old but have no significant symptoms. They are advised life style changes as advised below under 'Prevention'.

Medications. The bladder muscles can be relaxed and the prostate shrunken to some extent with medications. These are tried initially by the physician before any procedural treatment is adopted.

Minimally Invasive Procedures. Some treatments for prostate do not involve extensive surgery. **Trans Urethral Resection of Prostate**

(TUR-P) is one of the common procedures where an instrument is passed through the urethra and portions of the prostate are removed. This type of procedure may be done using Microwaves, Radiofrequency waves and Laser therapy.

Embolization. The blood supply to the prostate is cut off by injecting certain substances to block the artery which supplies the prostate. The blood supply to the prostate, when reduced, causes it to shrink in size and thereby relieve the symptoms.

Surgery. Surgery to remove the prostate is called Prostatectomy and is done when the prostate is very large and complications are present.

How can BPH be prevented.

Many lifestyle changes have been advised and are found effective in decreasing the chances of BPH developing in an individual. These are helpful in those who have minimal symptoms of BPH and are on treatment.

- Regular exercise has been found to decrease the chance of BPH in males. Any sort of aerobic exercise is advantageous.
- Reduction in the intake of alcohol and caffeine is important. Sugars and artificial sweeteners should be reduced.
- The patient is advised to reduce the intake of water and other fluids by evening so that night time urination is reduced.
- It is advisable for elderly individuals to empty their bladder before going out as they may not be able to find a toilet if they were to develop urgency to pass urine.
- Constipation should be avoided at all costs. Adequate fiber in diet and adequate water intake during day time are advised. If needed simple laxatives or stool softeners may be used.
- Certain medications used for depression, allergies, insomnia, and high blood pressure may worsen the symptoms of BPH. They are changed after requesting the physician.
- Patients with diseases like diabetes, high cholesterol or high

blood pressure should be careful to keep these under control.

- <u>Double voiding</u> is a technique advised when a patient has BPH. The patient is encouraged to relax and take time voiding urine. After passing urine, he should wait for 30-45 seconds and try passing urine again. Any residual urine in the bladder is thus expelled completely.

HERNIA

Hernia is a condition where an internal organ or tissue protrudes as a swelling through a weak area or the tissue covering it. For e.g., the intestines or fat inside the abdomen may push itself through the abdominal wall to be seen under the skin as a swelling. Hernia may also occur internally from one body space to another as in the stomach herniating into the chest cavity. This is an **Internal Hernia.**

The common sites where hernia occurs is the groin (**Inguinal Hernia**), Upper part of thigh (**Femoral Hernia**), through the belly button (**Umbilical hernia**) or the center of the abdomen (**Ventral Hernia**). The hernia occurring when the stomach protrudes into the chest cavity through the diaphragm is called the **Hiatus Hernia.**

A hernia may occur through a weak section of the abdominal wall or occur through a preexisting aperture in the abdominal wall which can enlarge over a period of time. A hernia can also occur in a scarred area in the abdomen as after a surgery. A scar in the abdominal wall is a weak area and a hernia occurs through it. Three-fourths of all hernias are either Inguinal or Femoral. Umbilical hernias are seen more in children where the belly button bulges out when the child cries, strains or coughs.

What are the Risk Factors causing hernia.

As a person grows old, the abdominal muscles weaken and the chances of hernia increase.

Women who have multiple pregnancies tend to develop hernias. Pregnancy by itself, is an important factor predisposing for the development of hernias.

Any condition which increases the pressure inside the abdomen frequently or permanently can lead to a hernia, e.g., Chronic cough as occurs in chronic lung disease, excess fluid inside the abdomen, tumors inside the abdomen.

Obesity is another important cause for hernias.

People who lift weights repeatedly also are at a risk of developing hernias.

What are the symptoms caused by Hernias.

The hernia is named depending on the site where it is found. The hernias of the abdominal wall are the commonest. Many of the hernias may have no symptoms in the early stages. But when they are large, they tend to produce symptoms.

- Often the hernia is seen as a collapsible swelling in the groin (inguinal hernia) or upper thigh (femoral hernia) or other areas. The swelling increases when the patient coughs or strains. In the male, the inguinal hernia may descend into the scrotum (the sac which holds the testicles). On feeling the swelling, it may feel 'dough-like' due to the intestines and/or fat within it.

- Some patients feel a dragging sensation or pain at the site of hernia.

- The swelling may totally disappear when the patient lies down and reappear on standing. The symptoms may increase after food.

- Hiatus hernias which occur internally can produce symptoms like heartburn, difficulty in swallowing or breathing difficulties. (See section on *GERD* under *Gastrointestinal Disorders*).

- Sometimes the intestines within the hernia can get strangulated leading to obstruction of passage of food through the intestines. This may cause nausea, vomiting, pain and bloating of the abdomen associated with severe constipation. This is an emergency which has to be treated surgically.

- Occasionally, when the opening through which the hernia protrudes is very narrow, it may cut off the blood supply to the intestines inside the hernia and this can lead to *gangrene* of the intestines. This is a very serious condition and needs immediate surgery.

How can Hernia be prevented.

Some of the important preventive aspects are.

- Maintenance of ideal body weight and avoiding obesity.
- Prompt treatment of chronic cough, constipation and other conditions which could lead to hernia.
- Avoiding smoking as it is a cause for cough.
- Regular exercise to strengthen the abdominal muscles in the adult will help the elderly preserve the muscular tone of the abdominal muscles in old age. The elderly should resort to aerobic exercises like walking, cycling, or swimming to keep up their muscular tone.
- Lifting heavy weights should be avoided as far as possible.

How are hernias treated.

In the early stages of hernia when symptoms are absent or mild, no active treatment is needed. The lifestyle modifications mentioned above suffice. When the hernia is causing symptoms, surgery is the only option.

Open surgery for the hernia is performed by opening the hernial sac, pushing the contents back into the abdomen and closing the hole through which the hernia bulges. This weak area may be reinforced using a synthetic mesh which prevents the hernia from reappearing.

Laparoscopic surgery ("Keyhole Surgery") is the modern method of surgery for hernias. The main advantage is that the hospital stay is reduced and the person can return to normal activities soon.

CERVICAL SPONDYLOSIS (CS)

The spine in the neck region is formed of seven vertebrae called the Cervical Vertebrae. Each vertebra is stacked on top of the other and joined by three small joints which contain cartilage. The bodies of the vertebrae are separated by shock-absorbing cartilages called **'Intervertebral Discs'**. The spinal cord is inside the canal formed by the stacked vertebrae and the nerves to the neck and upper arm arise from spinal cord and exit through the narrow spaces between the adjacent vertebrae. (See section on *Bone and Joints* – Book 1).

As one ages, changes occur in the vertebrae of the neck and their discs leading to stiffness and difficulty in movements of the neck. This condition is called **Cervical Spondylosis**. The cartilages of the discs become thinner and dry as one ages. The ligaments holding the vertebrae together become stiffer. The bones may grow small outgrowths called 'spurs' which may press on the nearby nerves and the spinal cord to produce further symptoms.

It is reported in many studies that by the age of 60 almost 80-85% of individuals have changes of CS in their neck vertebrae.

What are the Risk Factors which can cause CS.

There are a few risk factors which may make a person more susceptible to develop CS in middle age.

- Aging is the most important non-modifiable risk factor.
- Certain occupations where the person has to strain the neck by looking up constantly or keep the neck bent are important in the development of CS. Also, constant vibration of the body as in those who use the power drill can predispose to CS.
- Individuals who work on the computer with the screen kept above or below eyelevel thereby causing a strain on the neck can develop CS.
- Carrying heavy weights on the head as is seen in laborers in

Asian countries predisposes to the development of CS at a later age.

- Any injury to the neck like a fall or accident may lead to CS later in life.
- CS has been seen in certain families and is genetically related.

What are the symptoms of CS.

Most of the patients with CS during the early stages of the disease may be *asymptomatic*. The disease may be detected on routine examination or on a routine X-ray of the neck taken for other purposes.

Pain and stiffness of the neck is the commonest symptom which brings the patient to the doctor. The pain is more during movements of the neck.

Patients may feel a snapping, creaking or grating sound when the neck is moved.

The muscles of the neck may occasionally go into spasm causing a stiff neck with restriction of movements of the neck like turning the neck sideways or looking upwards.

Some patients feel dizziness, vertigo, or headache.

When the CS is severe, the bony spurs which are produced in the vertebrae may press on the nerves leaving the spinal cord to produce tingling and numbness in the upper limbs. Fine movements of the fingers may be affected and the handwriting of the patient may show changes. Occasionally, weakness of the upper limbs may be produced.

When the protruding intervertebral disc or bony spurs press on the spinal cord, the patient may have weakness of legs, difficulty in walking or problems with bladder or bowel control.

How is CS diagnosed.

CS is diagnosed by a careful clinical examination by the physician.

X-ray of the neck tells the physician the condition of the cervical vertebrae, the disc, and the presence of bony spurs.

Additional tests like CT scan, and MRI of the neck give more clear images of the changes in the vertebrae and discs and reveal any pressure on the nerves or the spinal cord.

Special tests like a *CT Myelogram* where a dye is introduced into the spinal canal and CT scan done shows the compression of the spinal cord. The function of the nerves in the upper limbs can be assessed using Nerve Function Tests.

How is Cervical Spondylosis treated.

There are many methods of treatment for CS. Patients with minimal symptoms may not need any treatment. Those with significant symptoms and restriction of neck movements are treated. The common methods of treatment are as follows:

Physical Therapy. This is done with the help of a Physical Therapist. The strength of the neck muscles are increased through various exercises. Stretching exercises are advised to increase the mobility of the vertebrae of the neck. Application of heat or cold to the neck to soothe pain and relieve stiffness is often helpful.

The patient is advised to maintain a proper posture. A thin pillow or cushion is used for the head at night while sleeping. While working on the computer, the person should take frequent breaks. The computer screen should be kept at eye level. Working in bed and sitting in a slouched posture while working must be avoided.

A soft collar or a brace may be provided by the physical therapist to be worn during the day time to ease the strain on the neck. It relieves the pain in the neck and the pressure on the nerves.

Medications. Pain relief is an important part of treatment and pain relieving medications are given. Medications are given to relax the neck muscles. Occasionally steroids are given to relieve the pain. Steroids may be injected into the neck to relieve the pain in CS. Severe pain may be relieved by injecting anesthetic agents to block the nerves.

Surgery. Surgery is done rarely in patients when there is pressure on the spinal cord leading to weakness in the lower limbs or bowel and bladder symptoms. It is done to relieve the pressure of a protruding disc or bony spur pinching the nerves to the upper arms.

How can one prevent CS in old age.

Some of the methods to prevent CS should be made part of the lifestyle of every young adult so as to avoid the condition in old age.

- Maintaining a good posture is of prime importance. Persons working with the computer need to take frequent breaks and avoid straining their neck by positioning the monitor at eye level.
- Regular exercise, including exercises of the neck is one of the best methods of prevention. Both strengthening and stretching exercises should be practiced. Simple aerobic and resistance exercises are important. Yogic exercises are good for the neck. _But certain contorted yogic postures should be avoided by the elderly as it can worsen the condition if they already have asymptomatic CS._
- One should be careful in young age and adulthood to prevent neck injuries while playing sports, exercising or during performance of hobbies like mountaineering, skiing, hiking etc.
- Carrying heavy weights on the shoulders or neck is risky.
- Slouching while sitting on the sofa or watching TV should not be done.
- One should not read with the head bent for long periods.. Breaks should be taken during any prolonged activity while using computers, reading, writing, knitting, stitching etc.

HEMORRHOIDS (PILES)

Hemorrhoids are also called Piles. They are enlarged and swollen veins which occur in the lower part of the rectum and the anus. They are bunches of veins like the varicose veins that occur in the legs. This is a disease which is likely to occur as one ages and is more common after the age of 50. It is reported that 1 in 20 Americans suffer from piles.

What causes Hemorrhoids.

Some of the causes which can lead to hemorrhoids are:

- Chronic constipation and diarrhea can lead to piles due to the constant strain of passing stools.
- Lifting of heavy weights as needed in some jobs.
- Obese persons have a propensity to develop piles.
- Some women develop piles during pregnancy.
- Unnecessary straining while passing stools is a frequent cause of hemorrhoids.

What are the symptoms of the disease.

The symptoms of hemorrhoids differ depending on whether they are outside in the anus or in the rectum inside.

- External piles may be felt as a soft swelling by the side of the anus.
- Internal piles produce a swelling inside the rectum. While passing stools, it may descend outside as a soft, spongy swelling only to return into the rectum at the end of bowel movement.
- Itching may be felt at the site of external piles.
- Bleeding may be seen while passing stools. Bright red blood may squirt into the toilet bowl at the end of passing stools.
- Pain and discomfort is felt by some individuals.

- Occasionally, the hemorrhoids may get inflamed and be very painful.
- At times, the blood within the piles may clot and it remains outside without going back into the rectum, leading to severe pain. (Prolapsed piles).
- Constant bleeding from the hemorrhoids can lead to anemia in the elderly patient and cause symptoms like fatigue and breathlessness.

It must be remembered that hemorrhoids may be a harbinger of the presence of cancer of the colon in some individuals and hence should not be ignored.

How is hemorrhoids diagnosed.

A simple clinical history and examination by the physician or surgeon can diagnose piles.

The doctor will examine the piles by introducing an instrument called *Proctoscope* or *Sigmoidoscope* into the rectum to look at the piles. He may also examine the piles by passing a gloved finger into the rectum to feel the pile mass.

How is Piles treated.

The important aspects of treatment are:

Lifestyle changes. An increase in fiber intake is one of the most important aspects of management of piles. A minimum of 25-30 grams of fiber should be taken daily. This prevents constipation and ensures adequate quantity of formed stools. If constipation is present, a stool softener or laxative may be taken at night. Water intake should be adequate. Regular exercise like walking is important in the elderly.

A Sitz bath is advisable. To take a sitz bath, a wide tub or basin is filled with warm water and a little salt added to it. The patient sits in the tub for about 15-20 minutes immersing the anus into the water. This can be done in a bathtub filling about 3 inches of warm water. The patient sits in it. Special Sitz bath bowls are available which can be placed on the top of the toilet bowl so that the patient can sit comfortably.

After the sitz bath, the area is patted dry and a hemorrhoids ointment is applied to the area. The ointment may be prescribed by the physician or in some countries it is available as an over-the-counter medication.

Medications. Severe pain may need pain relievers. Local application of ointments containing an anesthetic medication may be prescribed.

Minimally Invasive Procedures. Many types of minimally invasive procedures are available for the treatment of hemorrhoids. Injections of some chemicals can be done to shrink the piles. The piles can be surgically removed. Rubber band treatment is done where the stalk of the swelling is tightly bound by a rubber band so as to cut off its blood supply. The piles then shrinks and heals. Laser therapy and Electro-coagulation are other methods of treating hemorrhoids.

Surgery. The piles may be removed surgically by cutting and removing it. Another method of surgery is stapling the base of the pile mass using a stapler just like the one we use to staple papers together. The hemorrhoids shrinks away.

Prevention of Hemorrhoids.

Some of the preventive strategies are as follows.

- Adequate intake of Vegetables, Fruits, and Wholegrains to increase fiber in diet. Adequate water intake to prevent constipation.
- Regular exercise of which walking for 30-40 minutes a day is the best.
- Whenever there is an urge to pass stools, the individual should go to the toilet and pass stools and try not to withhold passing stools.
- Unnecessary straining should be avoided while passing stools.
- The person should maintain optimal body weight and avoid

obesity.
- Prolonged sitting is avoided to prevent piles.
- Passing stools should be made a routine daily morning habit after breakfast.

BACK PAIN

Back pain is one of the common causes of disability and absenteeism from work in modern times. It can vary from mild to severe debilitating pain in some individuals. As age increases, the chances of back pain increases. Back pain may be due to various disorders such as problems with the vertebral column, muscles of the back or due to diseases of internal organs like the kidneys.

What are the symptoms of Back Pain.

The pain is often in the mid and low back. It can vary from mild pain during movements or sitting to severe incapacitating pain. Occasionally the pain radiates down the leg. The pain increases on bending, twisting, walking, or standing.

When should medical attention be sought.

- Back pain lasting three or more weeks needs medical attention.
- Pain that is not relieved with rest.
- When the pain passes down into the legs, it indicates involvement of the nerves and should be investigated.
- Back pain associated with weight loss may indicate a serious disease.
- When bladder or bowel symptoms like difficulty in passing urine or constipation are associated, they should be investigated immediately.
- Fever associated with back pain should be investigated.
- Any back pain which begins after an accident, injury or a fall should be immediately checked to rule out fractures.
- When pain is associated with weakness of the legs or with numbness of the legs or the area around the buttocks.

What are the causes of back pain.

Some of the common causes of back pain in the elderly are:

1. <u>Muscular causes</u> like strain and sprain of ligaments can lead to back pain especially when lifting heavy weights or following unaccustomed activities.
2. <u>Diseases of the spine</u> like a degeneration of the intervertebral discs is a common cause in old age. The degenerated disc can protrude into the spinal canal and press on the spinal cord or on the nerves coming out of the spinal cord to produce pain or weakness of the lower limbs.
3. <u>Diseases of bones</u> like Osteoporosis, Osteoarthritis and various diseases of the joints causing arthritis can affect the joints in the spine leading to back pain.
4. <u>Awkward postures</u> can be a cause of muscular strain leading to back pain. Sitting for prolonged periods, standing for long periods, or using a mattress that does not support the back properly during sleep, can cause back pain.
5. <u>Infections</u> of the spine are an important cause of back pain.
6. <u>Diseases of internal</u> organs like kidney, liver or pancreas can present with symptoms of back pain. Cancer is a disease which may present with back pain when it involves the spine and vertebrae.
7. <u>Falls and minor accidents</u> in the elderly, can lead to back pain due to injury to the spine, ligaments, or muscle.
8. <u>Psychological stress</u> is an important factor which may present as back pain.

What are the Risk Factors that can lead to back pain.
Many risk factors are mentioned in the genesis of back pain.

- Age is an important factor. Back pain is seen more after the age of 40 though it can occur in the young too. The older the individual, the greater the chances of back pain.

- Overweight and obesity are risk factors for back pain.
- A sedentary lifestyle leading to weakness of the back and abdominal muscles poses a risk. Lack of exercise is an important risk.
- Smoking can reduce the blood flow to the spine and cause chronic cough both of which can cause back pain due to disc prolapse.
- People in certain occupations involving heavy lifting and bending are at a high risk of back pain.
- Arthritis of any type can cause back pain when the spine is involved.
- Psychological abnormalities like depression and anxiety may present as back pain in some individuals.

What are the diagnostic tests for back pain.

A thorough clinical examination by the doctor often reveals the cause of back pain.

Diagnostic tests like X-ray of the spine, CT scan and MRI scan are done when a detailed evaluation is needed. These reveal any fractures, diseases of the spine, disc, or muscles. Cancer of organs like the lungs, liver or breast may spread to the bones of the spine and are detected by these investigations.

Diseases like arthritis and infections are diagnosed by blood tests.

How is back pain treated.

The treatment of back pain depends on the cause. Any primary disease like cancer or arthritis causing back pain is managed accordingly.

The other methods of managing back pain are Physical Therapy, Medications and Surgical treatment.

Physical Therapy. Physical Therapy can be Active or Passive. In Passive physical therapy the patient is treated with hot or cold packs to relieve the symptoms of muscle spasm or strain.

Ultrasound stimulation of the back muscles relieves the pain in many individuals.

Transcutaneous Electrical Nerve stimulation (**TENS**) is used to relieve the pain. Here minor shocks are passed into the muscles of the back using electrodes fixed on the skin. This relieves the back pain.

The patient may be given supportive braces or corsets to support the back and relieve symptoms.

Physical massage of the back muscles relieves the pain and spasm of the muscles in some patients. Alternative therapy like *Ayurvedic* massage is helpful in such patients.

Occasionally, traction is given to the spine using weights to stretch the spine and thereby reduce pain in conditions like intervertebral disc prolapse.

Active physiotherapy with mild exercises and stretches are advised after the patient improves and the pain is relieved. This improves the muscle tone and strengthens them. This is a part of rehabilitation. Simple yoga exercises may be advised.

Acupuncture is an alternative method for pain relief.

Medications. Medications to relieve pain and relax the muscles are prescribed by the physician in appropriate cases. The medications are used for short periods only as prolonged use may cause side effects. Strong pain relieving drugs like opioids may be needed in some patients.

Antidepressant medications are given to some patients to reduce the symptoms.

Occasionally, injections of steroids are given around the spine to relieve the pressure and inflammation in the nerves.

Ointments and creams to relieve the pain are helpful in mild pain but may not be of much help in severe back pain.

Surgery. Various surgical procedures are available for treating back pain when the cause is primarily due to conditions in the spine. Surgery is needed to relieve the pressure on the nerves or spinal cord.

In disc prolapse, the offending prolapsed disc is removed surgically. Occasionally, part of the vertebra is removed or the adjacent vertebrae are fused together. Surgery is often resorted to only when other methods of relief fail.

How can back pain be prevented.

Preventing back pain is important especially in the elderly who are already affected by other co-existing diseases and weakening of muscles and bones. Furthermore, the elderly are prone for falls and accidents which are an important cause of back pain. Preventing falls in the elderly, hence, becomes a priority. (See section on *Falls in the Elderly – Book 1*).

The preventives strategies for back pain are as follows.

- Proper posture while sitting, walking, and sleeping are of utmost importance. One should sit erect with the back against the back of the chair. While sitting, it is always preferable to have a low back support with a small cushion or a rolled up towel. Ergonomic chairs with back support are available. It is important to sit erect with the feet flat on the floor. Slouching on chairs or on the sofa should be avoided. While sitting for long periods as in an office or in front of a computer, the knees and hips should be at the same level or the knees should be slightly at a higher level. A small footstool may be used to rest the feet. While sitting for long periods one should get up and walk every half an hour or so.

- Placing the laptop on one's lap while working makes one bend forward causing a strain on the back. The laptop should be placed on a desk with the screen at eye level. A mouse should be used preferably if working for long periods.

- One should not use the smart phone to text or watch videos for prolonged periods with the head and back bent. Reading, knitting, or stitching with the head bent forward is harmful.

- One should stand upright and not slouch while standing .

When one has to stand for long periods, the weight must be shifted between the legs alternatively. If possible, one foot may be placed on a small footstool alternatively while standing.

- When lying down to sleep, a firm mattress is important (neither too soft nor too hard). Sleeping on the back with a pillow below the knees relieves the strain on the spine. If the person prefers to sleep on the side, a pillow may be placed between the knees. _One should avoid sleeping prone on one's stomach._ The aim should be to get a comfortable sleep at night for at least 6-8 hours.

- Regular exercise like walking cycling or swimming are important to keep the abdominal and back muscles strong and flexible. Yoga is a good exercise to stretch and strengthen the muscles. _High impact exercises like jogging may not be ideal for the elderly as it can precipitate back pain in them._

- While lifting weights, one should squat down with the knees bent, hold the weight close to the body and then stand up slowly thus lifting the weight using the legs and not the back. _Keep the back straight and bend the knees only. Never bend down and lift a weight._ Avoid twisting movement while lifting a weight.

- While driving, especially for long distances, the seat should be adjusted so that the pedals are properly situated in front of the feet. During the drive frequent breaks should be taken and the individual should walk about for a few minutes before resuming driving.

- Proper footwear is important. High heels should be avoided as far as possible as they cause a strain on the back. Flat heels are ideal.

- Tight jeans should not be worn as it may interfere with bending and twisting. It is not advisable to carry a heavy wallet in the back pocket of one's pants. While driving one should not keep the wallet in the back pocket.

- When moving furniture, *pushing* is better than *pulling* them as it is easy on one's back.

- When carrying a hand bag, one with a long strap should be preferred and it should be worn across the chest with the strap on the opposite shoulder. This distributes the weight evenly. Avoid stuffing the handbag with too many things. A backpack should be worn straggling both shoulders, *never on one shoulder alone.*

- A balanced diet is important and adequate Vitamin D and Calcium should be available in the diet. The elderly may be given a Vitamin-Mineral supplement if the diet is insufficient in these nutrients.

- Smoking should be absolutely avoided to keep one's back healthy.

- Stress is an important causative factor in back pain and measures to reduce stress should be adopted.

FRAILTY

Frailty is defined as *"an age related syndrome of physiological decline characterized by marked vulnerability to adverse health outcomes."* [3]. With increasing age some individuals experience a gradual decline in function affecting multiple body systems causing a generalized decrease in, muscle strength, body weight, fitness and stamina. Frailty is often associated with one or more chronic diseases.

The prevalence of frailty in those over the age of 65 in the United States is reported to be 7-12%. In those aged 85 or above, it is seen in 25%, whereas it is only 3.9% in those in the age range of 65-74.

What causes Frailty.

Many causes are attributed to the development of frailty. One such cause is the decrease in the male and female hormones which occurs with age. This leads to a decrease in muscle mass in the body. Another cause propounded is chronic inflammation with a decline in immune function with a decrease in Vitamin D and increase in *Cortisol* in blood. Cortisol is a hormone produced by the adrenal gland and an increase denotes the presence of low grade inflammation in the body.

Frailty is caused by aging. But all elderly people are not frail. The importance of frailty lies in the fact that frail people have poor outcomes and increase in death rates when they develop any acute illness or have a surgical procedure. Frail individuals have a higher rate of hospitalizations and a higher risk for accidental falls leading to disability. Infections like Influenza, Covid-19 and Pneumonia can be fatal in a frail individual. Complications of any illness is increased in frail individuals and their dependency on others is more as independent living becomes difficult when one is frail.

How do you diagnose Frailty.

There are five characteristic criteria defined for Frailty. A person with <u>three of these five criteria,</u> is called frail. Frailty is more common in women and more in the Afro-Asian population. The five criteria are:

1. Unintentional Weight loss over 10 lbs or more in the past one year.
2. Physical exhaustion complained by the patient.
3. Muscle weakness as evidenced by a poor grip strength.
4. A slow speed of walking.
5. Low Physical Activity.

The importance of frailty is that decisions for active treatment of certain terminal illnesses are made in frail subjects with caution as the outcome is often not encouraging. Palliation is more important in these individuals rather than curative care.

When a person is diagnosed to have frailty the number of medications taken by the patient is often reviewed by the treating physician and only the absolutely essential ones are retained. All medications causing side effects are stopped. The dose of some medications as those used for diabetes or high blood pressure may have to be reduced lest the patient develop complications like low blood sugar or fall of blood pressure. The dictum of prescribing medication in frailty is always, **"*Start Low, Go Slow*"** in order to prevent side effects. The aim in a frail person is give him/her a better quality of life rather than a cure.

Resources

1. Prostate Enlargement. Benign Prostatic Hyperplasia. *National Institute of Diabetes and Digestive and Kidney diseases*. 2014.

https://www.niddk.nih.gov/health-information/urologic-diseases/prostate-problems/prostate-enlargement-benign-prostatic-

hyperplasia#:~:text=Benign%20prostatic%20hyperplasia%E2%80%94also%20called,pe
[1].

1. Frailty. Walston JD. *UpToDate* 2021.

https://www.uptodate.com/contents/
frailty#:~:text=Givens%2C%20MD%2C%20MSCE-,INTRODUCTION,vulnerabili
[2].

1. The Frailty Syndrome. Definition and Natural History. Qian-Li Xue. *Clinics in Geriatric Medicine*. 2011. 27: pages 1- 15.

https://www.ncbi.nlm.nih.gov/pmc/articles/
PMC3028599/#__ffn_sectitle

1. Adult Inguinal Hernia. Morrison Z et al. *Stat Pearls Publishing*. 2022.

https://www.ncbi.nlm.nih.gov/books/NBK537241/

1. Hemorrhoids. Perry KR et al. *Medscape* 2022.

https://emedicine.medscape.com/article/775407-overview

---

1. https://www.niddk.nih.gov/health-information/urologic-diseases/prostate-problems/prostate-enlargement-benign-prostatic-
hyperplasia#_853ae90f0351324bd73ea615e6487517__4c761f170e016836ff84498202b99827__853ae90f0351324bd73ea615e6487517_text_43ec3e5dee6e706af7766fffea512721_Benign_0bcef9c45bd8a48eda1b26eb0c61c869_20prostatic_0bcef9c45bd8a48eda1b26eb0c61c869_20hyperplasia_0bcef9c45bd8a48eda1b26eb0c61c869_E2_0bcef9c45bd8a48eda1b26eb0c61c869_80_0bcef9c45bd8a48eda1b26eb0c61c869_94also_0bcef9c45bd8a48eda1b26eb0c61c869_20called_c0cb5f0fcf239ab3d9c1fcd31fff1efc_periods_0bcef9c45bd8a48eda1b26eb0c61c869_20as_0bcef9c45bd8a48eda1b26eb0c61c869_20a_0bcef9c45bd8a48eda1b26eb0c61c869_20man_0bcef9c45bd8a48eda1b26eb0c61c869_20ages

2. https://www.uptodate.com/contents/
frailty#_853ae90f0351324bd73ea615e6487517__4c761f170e016836ff84498202b99827__853ae90f0351324bd73ea615e6487517_text_43ec3e5dee6e706af7766fffea512721_Givens_0bcef9c45bd8a48eda1b26eb0c61c869_2C_0bcef9c45bd8a48eda1b26eb0c61c869_20MD_0bcef9c45bd8a48eda1b26eb0c61c869_2C_0bcef9c45bd8a48eda1b26eb0c61c869_20MSCE-_c0cb5f0fcf239ab3d9c1fcd31fff1efc_INTRODUCTION_c0cb5f0fcf239ab3d9c1fcd31fff1efc_vulnerability_0bcef9c45bd8a48eda1b26eb0c61c869_20to_0bcef9c45bd8a48eda1b26eb0c61c869_20adverse_0bcef9c45bd8a48eda1b26eb0c61c869_20health_0bcef9c45bd8a48eda1b26eb0c61c869_20outcomes

1. 16 ways to avoid back pain. Smith MW. *WebMD* 2021

https://www.webmd.com/back-pain/tips-for-pain-relief

1. Back pain. Casiano VE et al. *Stat Pearls Publishing LLC* 2022

https://www.ncbi.nlm.nih.gov/books/
NBK538173/#_NBK538173_pubdet_

12. PALLIATIVE CARE & END OF LIFE CARE

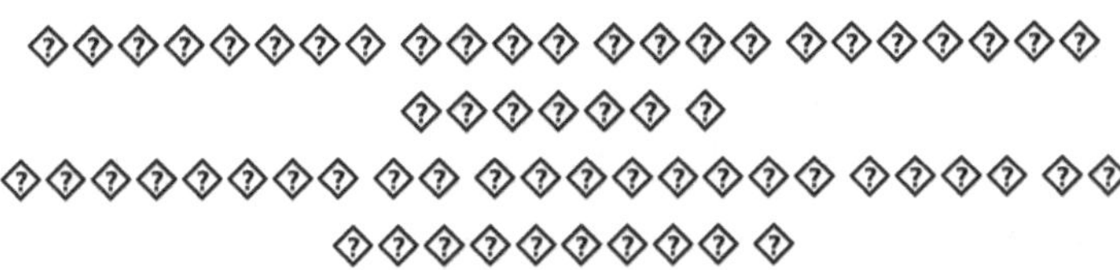

Anaayaasena maranam, Vinaa-dainyena jeevanam
Dehaantay tava saayujyam dehi may Parmeshvaram

Death without distress; A Life without affliction and dependence on others;

And when my soul leaves this body, I must only remember You; Grant me these O ! Lord.

The above verse is a common prayer on the lips of Hindus who are in the sunset years of life. The meaning is self-explanatory. End of Life is a difficult period for every individual when he or she needs comfort, solace, and support.

Palliative Care (PC) is the specialized care given to a person who has any incurable disease. It may be given alongside the curative treatment for the disease. In PC, only the symptoms of the patient are addressed. In addition, the patient receives psychological, social, and spiritual support. It is a holistic care of the patient.

End-of-Life care (EoL) on the other hand, denotes the support and medical care given to a dying person during the period near death – his last days. This could extend for day, weeks or rarely months. The care could be given at the home of the individual, in a hospital or hospice. EoL care is given to a person to make his death peaceful and comfortable.

PALLIATIVE CARE

Palliative Care (**PC**) is a specialized medical care that is given to patients with any serious incurable terminal illness like terminal Heart Diseases, Lung Diseases, Chronic Kidney Failure, Alzheimer's disease, Dementia or other Neurological diseases, and Terminal Cancer. The main aim of PC is to improve the quality of life of the patient and provide comfort. Concomitantly, treatment of the chronic disease is also continued.

Palliative Care is provided by a team of personnel consisting of doctors, nurses, social workers, nutritionists, and others. In PC only the symptoms of the patients are addressed. In addition, the patient is given social, emotional, and practical support. The family members also receive support during PC. It can be given at home, in a hospice, nursing home or hospital.

The World Health Organization in 2020 has stated that each year 56.8 million patients approximately need Palliative Care (PC). Of these 25.7 million are in their last year of life. But globally only 14% of those who need PC really get it.

It must be noted that Palliative Care and End-of-Life care are different. In PC, the patient simultaneously receives the definitive treatment for the illness like chemotherapy, radiation, dialysis, medications etc. Relief of symptoms, suffering and a holistic approach are the hallmarks of palliative care. PC is often provided when the life expectancy is usually less than six months. However, it can be extended further if the patient needs it. During End-of-Life care, palliative care is simultaneously continued.

Palliative care Management.

Pain. Pain management is the key factor in PC. Majority of patients with terminal cancer often have pain of variable intensity ranging from moderate pain to severe, intractable pain.

For control of pain, in mild cases simple pain relievers like Acetaminophen (Paracetamol) are used. Other medications like Ibuprofen, Diclofenac and Naproxen may be given. For more severe pain Opioid drugs may be used. They are Codeine, Tramadol and Morphine. Various other opioids are available. Morphine may be given orally as tablets or as injections. It must be given frequently.

Medications like steroids, anti-epileptic medications, and anti-depressant medications are used in pain relief, especially in pain due to terminal cancer.

Bone pain may need Radiotherapy. Pain due to muscle spasm, arthritis, or neurological diseases often needs Physical Therapy.

Other methods of pain relief which may be helpful are Acupuncture and **Transcutaneous Electrical Nerve Stimulation (TENS)** where a mild electrical current is passed through the skin to stimulate the nerves. The patient feels only a mild tingling feeling. This helps in relieving the pain of muscle spasm, arthritis, and nerve pain.

Pain always has a psychological component. Methods like Relaxation Therapy, Mindfulness Meditation, Yoga and Biofeedback are helpful in some patients.

In extreme cases, the nerves to the painful area can be blocked by injecting anaesthetic medications into the nerve to block the pain signals going to the spinal cord and brain. Rarely, the nerves are destroyed using chemicals, cold or heat. These are called *Ablation* procedures. They destroy the nerves permanently thereby relieving pain.

<u>Breathlessness</u>. Breathlessness is often a symptom which is distressing for both the patient and the relatives. Simple measures like propping up the patient in bed, using a humidifier in the room, keeping the windows open, or switching on a fan may relieve the symptom in many. Some patients feel relief on lying on the side rather than on their backs.

If the breathlessness is due to a specific medical cause, like fluid in the lungs, blockage due to sputum or secretions etc., it should be managed appropriately by the physician or nurse. Nebulization with medications will be needed in breathlessness due to asthma. Oxygen is needed for breathlessness only if the blood shows a low oxygen level. Otherwise administering oxygen will be redundant.

In some patients, anxiety may be the cause of breathlessness. In them simple anti-anxiety medications are helpful.

Digestive Problems. Some patients develop digestive problems like nausea or vomiting. These are treated with medications to prevent vomiting. Giving the patient small, but frequent meals substituting semi-solid food or liquid food, avoiding spicy foods and not resorting to force feeding of the patient, are simple measures which should be followed. If the nausea and vomiting are due to any of the medications which the patient is on, they should be discontinued or substituted with others.

Constipation is not uncommon in patients who are in bed. Adequate fluid intake and adequate fiber in diet helps in reducing constipation. A gentle laxative may be given to them at bedtime to ease passing motion in the morning. A bedside commode should be provided.

Anxiety and Depression. Anxiety and depression are common in patients with an incurable illness as they are aware of the inevitability of death. The physician will prescribe medications for anxiety or depression after assessing the patient.

Dehydration. Dehydration should be prevented in the patient by ensuring adequate fluid intake. The patient must be encouraged to drink water or other fluids frequently. _Alcohol must be avoided_. If the patient is unable to drink due to problems in swallowing, he may need intravenous fluid or be given tube feeding.

Care of the Skin. The care of the skin is important in preventing the development of complications like bed sores. The skin should be kept clean and moisturized. Sponge baths may be given for those who cannot bathe themselves. A lip balm should be applied to the lips to prevent drying. Frequent sips of water help in preventing dry mouth. Bed sores should be avoided by frequently changing the posture of bedridden patients. A special Air mattress may be provided to prevent bed sores. (See section in *Bed Sores in Book 1*).

<u>Emotional & Spiritual Needs</u>. The PC team also helps the patient in their emotional and spiritual needs. The patients on PC are often apprehensive regarding the outcome of their illness. The team helps them to understand their problems and helps them overcome the anxiety and fear of the terminal illness. Talking to the patients and allowing them to air their concerns and fears is a simple way of setting their minds at ease. The simple act of holding hands or massaging are important aspects of palliative care where the patient feels relaxed and relieved.

Reading to the patient is often helpful in keeping the patient engaged and at the same time relieving the feeling of loneliness, boredom, and depression.

Spiritual needs of patients are met by arranging a chaplain or any other religious person like an Imam, Rabbi, Swamiji, or a Priest to visit the patient. The patient is encouraged to read books and religious texts as per his / her inclination. Listening to soothing music and religious discourses on the internet or from recorded speeches helps them. Simple religious hymns and *slokas* are soothing to listen to. Each patient is given the choice depending on his religion and belief in choosing the appropriate spiritual guidance.

Even when patients are unconscious terminally, (*coma*) they are still able to hear and comprehend what is going around them. This state is called "**Coma Vigil**" in medical parlance. The patient can understand what others around him are saying though he cannot respond. *Hence, it is very important that the relatives and visitors be careful of what they speak in the presence of a person who is unconscious.*

END OF LIFE CARE

Death is not the opposite of life, but a part of it – Haruki Murakami *"End-of-life care is the term used to describe the support and medical care given during the time surrounding death."* This is the definition provided by the *National Institute of Aging*. It aims to keep the person physically, mentally, and emotionally comfortable during his/her last days. Only 10-15% of people are blessed with a sudden death with minimum distress.

It has been found that in Western countries, artificial life support gets withdrawn <u>with consent</u> in 90% of patients who are at end of life. Unfortunately, in some developing countries like India it happens only in about 22% of individuals. In countries like India, the patient does not have the freedom to choose the End-of-life care that he desires and leaves it to the discretion of his relatives and children. Consequently, the patient is put to much distress in the hospital during his last days without having a say in the treatment. Withdrawal of treatment in the last days is often not acceptable to the relatives as they express the willingness to *"try everything possible"* for the patient and end up blaming the doctor and the hospital when the patient dies! The concept of End-of-Life Care still has to catch on in some societies.

The awareness regarding importance of E-o-L care is more in the Western world and patients are already prepared for a peaceful death and have opted to avoid unnecessary procedures and interventions terminally. Dying lonely in an Intensive Care facility surrounded by gadgets and tubes rather than in the presence of well-meaning and warm-hearted near and dear ones is a bête noire of any individual. But it does remain a sad fact today in many societies. Some relatives are so obsessed with prolonging life, that they blame the doctors who suggest that 'nothing more can be done'. Confrontation and altercations by relatives of patients *in extremis* is not unknown many countries like India.

"The Quality of Death is as important as the Quality of Life."

Death is unpredictable. End-of-Life care (EoL) aims at helping the patient have a peaceful and dignified death. No doctor can predict when a patient will die. But in most cases, the final days can be determined. The E-o-L care may extend from days to weeks and occasionally more. The most important concerns at this time would be mitigating the symptoms of the patient and relieving the anguish of the patient and family.

Medications which are therapeutic, and curative may be withdrawn at this stage. However, pain relieving medications are continued. If the patient is unable to drink fluids, intravenous fluids may be given at the discretion of the physician. Tube feeding is done if needed.

In the management of a patient during E-o-L, the wishes of the family is of prime importance. The patient may or may not be involved in this decision. The decisions should be based on individual merits of the case and generalizations cannot be followed here.

Charles Garfield in his article, *"Seven Keys to a Good Death"* [6] describes the important features of a 'Good Death' where the person has no pain, he has resolved his interpersonal conflicts, his wishes are satisfied, he has handed control of his possessions to a trusted person and has decided to avoid all unnecessary procedures and life sustaining treatment.

All the particulars discussed in the section on Palliative Care of the patient are applicable in E-o-L care also. The patient should be made as comfortable as possible. Pain should be relieved. Any wishes of the conscious patient should be respected and carried out. It is ideal for the family members to be present at the bedside of the dying patient during the last days. An endeavour should be made to provide solace to the patient. Simple handholding by a near and dear one gives great comfort and relief to the sinking patient.

All investigations which are not essential are stopped. Antibiotics are not necessary at this stage. Curative medications are not given at this stage. The family should be told about this plan of care in advance to prevent misunderstanding and complaints later.

A decision regarding Resuscitation should be made. Mostly patients would have expressed their willingness regarding resuscitation or mechanical ventilation prior to falling seriously ill. (See section on *Living Will* below). In some countries, the **Do Not Resuscitate** (**DNR**) order can be given by the doctor depending on the patient's previously conveyed wishes. Often this is given in writing by the patient well in advance.

However, in some countries like India, where the concept of the "*Living Will*" is not widely accepted or popular yet, this is not possible. This is an ethical dilemma often for the treating physician and the family and the close relatives must be apprised of all the details of the disease and the unfavourable outcome. Proper communication is of prime importance in this scenario to avoid distress to the families and complaints later. The legal aspects of this must be discussed in each case before a decision is taken. The legal aspects and mandates on "Passive Euthanasia" vary from country to country.

How to recognize that a patient is dying.

A dignified and peaceful death is what everyone would like to have. A person is said to have 'died well' if he did not feel significant pain or psychological distress during his last days. Both the caregivers and relatives should understand that the patient is dying. Some of the pointers that a person is dying are as follows.

- The patient may turn mute and withdrawn. He may stop conversing and sink into a state of drowsiness with fits of sleep and awakening. Occasionally patients lose consciousness towards the end.
- Some persons may become confused and not recognize their kith and kin towards the end. Some persons may see visions of people who are not present near them.
- They may become unable to feed due to loss of appetite.

Swallowing may be impaired.

- The breathing pattern may change and become shallow or irregular. The patients may have periods when breathing stops only to recover again with a gasp.
- Some individuals lose control of their bladder and bowel and may become incontinent.
- The urine quantity may become reduced, and it may be concentrated and dark in color.
- Often the skin turns cool, and the extremities become clammy and develop a bluish color due to reduction in blood circulation in the tissues.
- Some patients may develop involuntary movements of their fingers or toes and seem to pick at the bed linen. They may be restless or delirious towards the end and become irritable.
- The blood pressure of the patient drops towards the end and the limbs may become limp and flaccid.
- Some have secretions and saliva accumulated in the throat and chest leading to a rattling sound often referred to as the '*death rattle*'. This is distressing for the relatives around the patient.

During this period, when it is certain that the patient is approaching the end of his life, all the curative treatment is withdrawn, and the patient is given only supportive management to keep him/her comfortable. If there are secretions in the throat and chest, the doctor may remove them or prescribe medications to dry them up. If pain is still a problem, morphine or other opioid medications are given.

LIVING WILL AND ADVANCE DIRECTIVES

The **Living Will and Advance Directives** for Medical Decisions are legal documents which give instructions as to what medical care should be given to a person if he cannot decide for himself as in an unconscious patient or extreme dementia. A person can make a living will in advance leaving instructions on what treatment he should receive and what should not be done if he is not capable of taking that decision due to incapacity or inability to communicate. These are instructions to medical personnel in case of terminal illnesses, accidents or dementia regarding End-of-Life care needed by the patient.

'Passive Euthanasia' is a term used to indicate the withholding of life-sustaining treatment like ventilation, tube feeding or CPR in the best interests of the patient and '*allowing the person to die*' rather than keeping him alive. This is a highly emotive decision to be taken by the patient's near and dear ones and is a highly debatable topic.

The Black's Law Dictionary defines an **Advance Medical Directive** as "*a legal document explaining one's wishes about medical treatment if one becomes incompetent or unable to communicate*".[Ref. 7]

In this document, a spouse, an adult child, a family member, a friend, or any other person is mentioned, who can take the decision on behalf of the incapacitated patient. *The patient's doctor cannot be named to take the decision*. This document is prepared in advance by the patient when he is healthy and in a position to take sensible decisions. This is a Medical or Health Care Power of Attorney.

The living will specifies what treatment the patient should or should not receive if he himself is unable to take the decision for himself. Decisions regarding mechanical ventilation to prolong life, pain management and donation of an organ or the whole body for medical research purposes etc., are mentioned in the living will.

The starting of Cardiopulmonary Resuscitation (CPR), mechanical ventilation, tube feeding, dialysis, use of antibiotics, organ donation and palliative care are included in the living will. A decision not to Resuscitate known as *"Do Not Resuscitate"* (**DNR**) is also mentioned in the will.

The Living Will and Advance Directives are legal documents which are notarized. The original copy is kept by the patient in an easily accessible location known to the relatives. A copy is given to the hospital or the doctor treating the patient. The document can be reviewed and changed, if necessary, by the patient later if he develops a new disease or if the document is more than 10 years old.

In India, however, the Living Will and Advance directives are not practical as there is no clear-cut law yet regarding this. According to Professor M. R. Rajagopal, Chairman of Pallium India, *"...advanced medical directives will be valid. But the Supreme Court also laid down a condition that such directives will have to be countersigned by a judicial magistrate of the first class."* [5]. This is a cumbersome procedure and very difficult for the families of the patient to comply.

The Supreme court in India is hearing the case as of January 2023 and is favourably inclined to remove the cumbersome clauses in its previous guidelines issued in 2018 and modify the guidelines to make the procedure simpler and make the Living Will practical possibility. [9]

It is preferable if the person carries a copy of the Living Will while traveling. A small card indicating the contact person and the telephone number should always be carried by the person in his wallet.

It must be noted that the Living Will is different from the Last Will and Testament of a person which comes into effect *only after the death of the person* and is related to the physical assets and possessions of the person.

"Netherlands was the first country to allow euthanasia and assisted suicide in 2002. Belgium followed suit as the second country to legalize

euthanasia in the same year. Luxembourg, Australia, New Zealand, Spain, Austria, Colombia, and Canada permit voluntary euthanasia. Canada may soon expand the purview of its law allowing euthanasia to include people suffering from mental health conditions. Assisted suicide is permissible in Germany, Switzerland, and some states of the United States (California, Washington DC, Oregon, Vermont, Montana, and Colorado). All these countries have prescribed stringent rules under which euthanasia is permitted." [9].

It has been estimated that 45% of Americans had a Living Will in 2020.

Resources

1. Davidson's Principles and Practice of Medicine. 23rd ed. Elsevier. 2018. Chapter 34. *Pain and Palliative Care.* Pages 1337-1356.

2. Care of Dying Adults in the Last Days of Life. *National Institute for Health Care and Excellence (NICE) Guideline* 2015.

https://www.nice.org.uk/guidance/ng31/ifp/chapter/
About-this-information

3. Role of Palliative Care at the End of Life. Rome RB et al. *The Ochsner Journal.* 2011. 11 : pages 348-352.

https://www.ncbi.nlm.nih.gov/pmc/articles/PMC3241069/

4. Compassionate End Of Life Care: Needed Focus On Suffering. Geriatrics & Gerontology Initiative: International Workshop on Care of the Elderly. Rajagopal MR. *BMH Medical Journal.* 2020. 7(Suppl) pages S 8 – 13

https://www.babymhospital.org/BMH_MJ/index.php/BMHMJ/
article/view/242

5. Prof. M.R. Rajagopal, Chairman Pallium India, Trivandrum (*Personal Communication*).

6. Living Wills and Advance Directives for Medical Decisions. *Mayo Clinic Staff.* 2022.

https://www.mayoclinic.org/healthy-lifestyle/consumer-health/in-depth/living-wills/art-20046303

7. Seven Keys to a Good Death. Charles Garfield. *Greater Good Magazine.* 2014.

https://greatergood.berkeley.edu/article/item/seven_keys_to_good_death.

8. Living Will – A Partial Way. Ankush Saraf. *Legal Service India E-Journal.* 2022.

https://www.legalserviceindia.com/legal/article-1116-living-will-a-partial-way.html

9. Dr Veena Aggarwal, Consultant Women's Health, CMD and Editor-in-Chief, IJCP Group & Med talks Trustee, Dr KK's Heart Care Foundation of India 25 January 2023

https://www.emedinexus.com/post/35460/

* * * * * * * * * * * * *

A Humble Request to the Reader

Thank you for buying and reading this book. May I request your indulgence for one more favour.

I hope you enjoyed reading this book and derived benefit from the various topics discussed.

Kindly give your sincere and valuable review of this book in the Amazon site. Your rating and candid review will be a great inspiration and encouragement to me.

I would also request you to check my other two books – *Tell Me a Story, Grandpa* and *Grandpa Tell Me More Stories* which are a compilation of short stories with morals, mainly written with children in mind.

Also, the book of '*In Search of a Bridegroom*' is an interesting Autobiographical Fiction which will be of great interest to the reader.

Do not forget to read the Book 1 in this series titled 'How to Face the Health Challenges While Growing Old'. The two books form the two volumes on *Problems of the Elderly*.

You can contact me at my email address kvsauthor@gmail.com

https://www.linkedin.com/in/sahasranam-dr-k-v-3231a13a/ (Linked In)

https://medium.com/@ramani2911/membership (Medium.com)

https://www.amazon.com/author/sahasranamkalpathy

(Amazon Author Central)

GLOSSARY

Abdomen The part of the body containing the digestive organs, kidneys etc. Above, it is bound by the diaphragm separating it from the chest and below, by the pelvis.

Ablation The removal or destruction of a body part or tissue, or its function.

Accommodation The ability of the eye to change the curvature of the lens to focus the image on the retina.

Acute Intense : Severe : Of a sudden onset.

Allergen Any substance that causes an allergic reaction.

Anti-coagulant A medicine used to prevent blood clots. Used in Stroke and Heart Attacks.

Antioxidants A substance rich in Vit. C, E, or other organic compounds that remove the harmful oxidizing agents in a living organism.

Anus The opening at the end of the alimentary canal through which waste products after digestion (stools) are expelled.

Apnea Temporary cessation of breathing, especially during sleep.

Appendix A small worm-like structure attached to the beginning of the large intestines (cecum), opening into it.

Asymptomatic Producing or showing no symptoms.

Atopic Dermatitis Eczema : Itchy, Dry skin with inflammation.

Atrophy Wasting away or degeneration of cells in a tissue.

Autoimmune diseases Diseases where the body's own immune system attacks the healthy cells in the body.

Ayurveda A traditional Hindu system of medicine where treatment is by herbs, diet, massage and breathing exercises. It is an alternative system of medicine common in India.

Benign Not harmful : Not cancerous.
Bhajan A Hindu devotional song

Biopsy Removal of cells or tissues to study in the laboratory regarding the nature of the illness. E.g., biopsy of liver to detect diseases.

Blister A fluid filled sac in the outer layer of skin.

Buttermilk A slightly sour liquid remaining after butter has been churned and removed from curd.

Candida albicans It is a fungus that is normally found in the mouth, intestines etc., but causes infection when the body's defenses are down.

Carbohydrates The group of organic compounds which include sugars, starches, and cellulose.

Catatonia An abnormal mental state in psychiatric diseases causing abnormal behaviour and movement. The person may sit or assume a fixed position for long periods. Seen in Schizophrenia.

Cecum A pouch like structure at the beginning of the large intestines where the small intestines joins.

Cervix The lower narrow end of the uterus which forms a canal between the cavity of the uterus and the vagina.

Chapati A thin pancake of unleavened whole-grain bread cooked on a griddle or pan.

Circadian Rhythm Physical, mental and behavioral changes that follow a 24-hour cycle in humans and animals.

Clitoris An erectile small organ in the vulva of female and is associated with sexual arousal.

Cold Sore Tiny fluid-filled blisters around the mouth seen during fever, due to Herpes simplex virus infection.

Coma A deep unconsciousness that lasts for a long period usually due to an injury to or disease of the brain.

Co-morbidities The simultaneous presence of two or more diseases in a person.

Compulsion An irresistible urge to behave in a particular way against one's conscious wishes.

Computerized Tomography Scan (CT scan) A series of X-rays which is converted by the computer into a composite picture which is two or three dimensional.

Conjunctiva The mucous membrane that lines the front of the eye and the inside of the eyelids.

Constrict Become Narrow : Narrowing (constriction) of blood vessels due to the muscles in their walls.

Cornea The glass-like transparent layer in front of the eye through which light passes into the eye.

Cortisol A hormone secreted by the Adrenal gland.

CPR **C**ardio **P**ulmonary **R**esuscitation. It is a life-saving technique of Heart compression and breathing given to a person who has a cardiac arrest.

Crown The exposed part of the tooth that is covered with enamel.

Cryotherapy The use of extreme cold in medical treatment or surgery.

Culture The growth of microorganisms like bacteria, viruses, or fungus in the laboratory.

Curettage Removal of tissue by scraping using a spoon-shaped instrument (Curette) with sharp edges.

Cuticle It is the fold of skin seen at the bottom edge of the finger nail.

Cytokine A protein made by the body which affects the immune system.

Decubitus Ulcer Bed sore.

Dental Caries Tooth Decay.

Dermatologist A medical practitioner specialized in diagnosing and treating skin diseases.

Dialysis A procedure to remove waste products and excess fluid from the blood in kidney failure.

Dilation & Curettage (D&C) A surgical procedure where the cervix of the uterus is dilated and the interior of the uterus curettaged (scraped) to remove tissues for diagnosis or treatment.

Dilate To make or become wider, open, or larger.

Diverticular disease A condition where small pouches or pockets (Diverticula) develop in the wall of the large intestine.

Diverticulitis Infection and inflammation in the Diverticula in the large intestines.

Diverticulosis The condition where multiple Diverticula are present in the Large intestines : Diverticular disease.

DNA Deoxyribo **N**ucleic **A**cid is the hereditary material present in all chromosomes and is the self-replicating material present in all organisms.

Downs Syndrome A set of cognitive and physical symptoms produced in a patient due to abnormality in Chromosome-21 of the patient where an extra copy of chromosome is present. (3 chromosomes).

Duct A tube or vessel in the body through which fluids like secretions and excretions pass.

Dysgeusia A distorted sense of taste : Bad taste in the mouth.
Dysphagia Difficulty or discomfort during swallowing.

Eczema A skin condition where patches of skin become thick and inflamed often with blisters and itching sensation.

Electroconvulsive Therapy A procedure done under anesthesia where small electric currents are passed through the brain for treatment purposes.

Electrolyte A substance which has a positive or negative charge when dissolved in water. E.g., Sodium, Potassium, Calcium.

Electrophoresis The movement of a charged particle through a fluid or gel under the influence of an electric field.

Emollient A substance that soothes and softens the skin.

Emulsification The process of breaking down large fat globules into tiny particles for easy digestion.

Encephalitis Inflammation of the brain due to infections or allergic causes.

Endometrium The inner lining of the cavity of the uterus.

Endoscope An instrument introduced into the body to view the internal organs or parts.

Enema A procedure where liquid is introduced into the rectum to evacuate its contents (stools) and also to introduce medications.

Enzyme A substance produced by the body which catalyzes a biochemical reaction.

Erectile Dysfunction Inability of a male to maintain an erection to achieve a satisfactory sexual activity.

Erythropoietin A hormone secreted by the kidneys which helps in increasing the production of red blood cells.

Esophagoscopy Examining the interior of the esophagus using an instrument (Esophagoscope) by passing it into the esophagus through the mouth.

Esophagus The tube-like part of the Alimentary Canal that connects the mouth to the stomach : Gullet.

Estrogen Hormones in the female which produce the female characteristics in a body.

Exfoliation Removing dead skin cells from the outer layer of skin.

Fats Oily or greasy substances produced by the body and stored in fat cells under the skin and elsewhere in the body : A chemical composed of Glycerol and Fatty acids.

Fecal impaction A mass of thick dry stools that cannot be passed out of the rectum normally and gets lodged there.

Feces Waste matter excreted after digestion : Excrement : Stools : Poop.

Fetus The developing human form within the uterus from eight weeks to birth.

Flavonoids Plant pigments which have health benefits as they have antioxidant properties.

Freckles Small patches light brown in color usually occurring on the face and increasing by exposure to the sun.

Gangrene Localized death of tissue in a living body, usually caused by lack of blood supply and/or infection.

Gastric Cancer Cancer the stomach.

Gastroenterologist A medical practitioner specialized in the diagnosis and treatment of the diseases of the Gastrointestinal tract and allied organs.

Gingivitis Inflammation of the gums in the mouth.

Gluten A protein found in grains like Wheat, Barley, and Rye. It gives the elastic character to dough. Some people are allergic to it.

Gynecologist A medical practitioner specialized in diagnosing and treating diseases of the female reproductive system.

Hair Follicle The sheath of cells and tissue that covers the root of the hair.

Helicobacter pylori A bacterium that causes inflammation and ulcers in the stomach and intestines.

Hemoglobin A red protein present in the Red blood cells in blood concerned with transporting oxygen and carbon dioxide to and from lungs to tissues.

HIV/AIDS Human Immunodeficiency Virus which attacks the immune system of humans to cause Acquired Immunodeficiency Syndrome and destroys the immune cells so that the patient becomes prone to infections.

Homeostasis A state of physiological balance of all systems in the body needed for the body to survive and function normally.

Human intestinal microbiota The various microorganisms normally present in the intestines is collectively called so.

Hymen A membrane which partly closes the opening of the vagina in virgins.

Hypercalcemia Calcium level in blood above normal.

Hyperplasia An enlargement of a tissue or organ caused by increased multiplication of cells in it.

Hypothermia It is a dangerous condition where the body loses heat leading to core temperature below 35°C or 95°F, usually due to cold exposure.

Hysterectomy Surgical operation to remove part or whole of uterus.

Hysteroscope An instrument used to look at the interior of the uterus.

Hysteroscopy The procedure of looking into the uterus using a Hysteroscope.

Immunocompromised A condition where the immune systems are weak, unable to fight external invasion by infectious agents.

Immunoglobulin Proteins present in blood which function as Antibodies.

Immunosuppressant drug A drug which decreases the body's immune responses.

In extremis Near Death : At the point of death : At an extremely difficult situation.

Infection The entry and growth of microorganisms into the body causing harm to the body.

Infestation The presence of large number of insects or parasites in the body. They may be external like lice or mites or internal like intestinal worms.

Inflammation A physical condition where a part of the body becomes red, swollen, painful and warm, often as a result of an infection or injury.

Insomnia Inability to sleep : A habitual Sleeplessness.
Intimacy Closeness : Close familiarity or friendship.

Intraocular Lens (IOL) A lens implanted in the eye as a part of treating cataract or severe short-sightedness.

Itch mite A parasitic mite that burrows into the skin to cause an itchy skin disease called Scabies.

Jet Lag A temporary sleep problem occurring in persons traveling across several time zones.

Kegels Exercises Exercises to strengthen the pelvic floor muscles which support the uterus, bladder, rectum, and small intestines.

Laparoscopic Surgery "Keyhole Surgery" : An instrument called Laparoscope is passed into the abdomen or pelvis through a small hole in the abdominal wall to see the inside of the abdomen or pelvis and perform surgery without causing a large wound as in conventional surgery.

Lesion An area of abnormal tissue in the body. E.g., Ulcer, Tumor, Abscess.

Lymph The colorless fluid present in the lymphatic system containing white blood cells that fight infections.

Lymph node A bean shaped small organ located along the lymph channels containing white blood cells (Lymphocytes) which fight infections.

Lymphocyte A type of white blood cell seen in the lymphatic system and lymph nodes concerned with fighting infections.

Magnetic Resonance Imaging (MRI) Use of magnetic field and computer generated radio waves to create images of organs in the body and used in the diagnosis of diseases.

Masala A blend of spices used in Indian cuisine.

Melanin The dark brown to black pigment present in the hair, skin, and Iris of the eye.

Melanocyte Specialized cells in the skin which form the pigment Melanin that gives color to the skin, hair, and iris of the eye.

Menopause Cessation of menstruation, usually between the age of 45 and 50.

Menstruation The process in which a woman discharges the blood and tissue from the uterine lining (Endometrium) every month starting from puberty till menopause.

Metabolism The chemical changes that occur in the cells in the body converting food into energy.

Metastasis The spread of cancer cells from their initial site of origin to other parts of the body.

Microorganism An organism seen only through a microscope like bacteria, viruses, and fungi.

Moisturizer A lotion or cream used to prevent dryness of the skin and retain moisture.

Mucus A thick slimy substance secreted by the lining membranes of many organs like nose, mouth, lungs, and gut.

Mucus Membranes The moist inner lining of body cavities and organs which secrete mucus. E.g., Lung, Mouth, Nose, Stomach.

Mutation Change in the structure of a DNA causing a change in the gene.

Myelogram A diagnostic test done to detect problems in the spinal cord. It is done by injecting a dye into the spinal canal and taking X-rays.

Myopia Near sightedness : Short sightedness : Distant objects appear blurred.

Nephrologist A medical practitioner specialized in the diagnosis and treatment of diseases of the Kidneys.

Neutrophil A type of white blood cell which is concerned with fighting infection by invading microorganisms.

Nit The egg of a head louse. It is attached to the hair.

Norwegian Scabies A severe form of scabies that occurs with crusted lesions in the skin seen in severely weak or immunocompromised persons.

NSAID Non-Steroidal Anti-Inflammatory Drug. A type of medications prescribed commonly for pain like joint pains.

Obsession A thought or idea that keeps on intruding the mind of a person with inability to stop that thought.

Oncologist A medical practitioner specialized in the diagnosis and treatment of cancer.

Ophthalmologist A medical practitioner specialized in the diagnosis and treatment of diseases of the eye.

Optic nerve The nerve that carries signals from the retina of the eye to the brain.

Optometry The profession of examining the eye for visual defects and prescribing corrective lenses.

Oral Thrush A fungal infection in the lining of the mouth caused by the fungus – Candida albicans.

Orbit The socket in front of the skull holding the eyeball.

Pallor A condition where the person appears pale and his skin and mucous membranes are lighter than usual in color.

Pediculosis Infestation of the hairy parts of the body or clothing with the eggs, larvae, or adults of lice. E.g., Head Lice.

Peptic ulcer disease A sore or ulcer in the lining of the esophagus, stomach, or intestines.

Peristalsis A wave like involuntary contraction of the muscles of the intestines and gut causing food to be pushed forward.

Peritoneum A thin membrane that lines the inner aspect of the abdomen and covers most of the abdominal organs.

Peritonitis Infection of the peritoneum usually due to bacterial invasion.

Pessary A solid device made of silicone which is inserted into the vagina to act as a support for the uterus. Medicated pessaries containing contraceptive and other medications are used.

Photocoagulation The use of Laser beam or other intense light source to coagulate and destroy a small area of tissue, usually in the retina.

Plaque A sticky and slimy substance containing bacteria that collects on teeth and produced teeth decay.

Plasma The clear yellowish liquid part of the blood that contains the blood cells and proteins in it.

Polyp A small growth, often benign with a stalk arising from the mucous membrane as in the large intestines.

Polysomnography Sleep Study : A detailed test to diagnose sleep disorders where brain waves, oxygen in blood, heart rate, breathing and other parameters are monitored.

Pore A tiny opening in the surface of the skin or mucous membrane through with gases or liquids can pass out.

Positron Emission Tomography (PET scan) An imaging technique where isotopes are used to reveal the biochemical and metabolic functions of tissues and organs.

Post Herpetic Neuralgia Residual pain occurring in areas of skin which had shingles.

Pranayama The control of breath in Yoga through breathing exercises.

Presbyopia Farsightedness or Longsight caused by loss of elasticity of the lens of the eye in old age. Near vision is defective.

Probiotic Live microorganisms or their spores used as dietary supplements to help digestion and normal bowel function.

Proctoscope An instrument used to examine the insides of the rectum.

Progesterone A steroid hormone released by the ovary which prepares the uterus for pregnancy.

Prolapse Displacement of an organ or a part of it downwards usually protruding through an orifice. E.g., Uterus Prolapsing into vagina.

Prophylaxis Action taken to prevent disease. E.g., Vaccination.

Proteins An organic compound formed of Amino Acids. They are an essential part of all of the body organs.

Psoriasis A skin disease with red, scaly, itchy patches.

Pupil The round hole in the center of the Iris of the eye which permits light to enter the eye.

Remission A decrease or disappearance of signs and symptoms of a disease like cancer.

Repetitive Transcranial Magnetic Stimulation A noninvasive procedure using magnetic fields to stimulate brain cells in depression.

Retina The layer of light sensitive cells at the back of the eye that receives light and converts it into signals to be sent to the brain through the Optic Nerve.

Retinal detachment A condition where the thin layer of cells of the retina separates from its attachment to the eye and becomes loose.

Root The part of a human body like Nail, Tooth or Hair that is buried underneath the skin or other tissues like the gums.

Saline A solution of common salt and water. Normal Saline indicates a 0.9% solution of Sodium Chloride.

Sarcoptes scabiei The parasitic mite that causes Scabies in humans.
Satsang A spiritual discourse or a religious gathering.

Scabicide A medication used to treat Scabies. That which kills the mites.

Serum The amber colored, protein rich fluid which separates when blood clots.

Sexuality The capacity for sexual feelings : Sexual Orientation of a person.

Sigmoid colon The 'S' shaped last part of the large intestines which joins the Rectum.

Sigmoidoscope A flexible tube inserted through the anus to view the rectum and sigmoid colon.

Sloka A couplet of Sanskrit verse chanted as a prayer.

Spasm A sudden involuntary contraction of muscle in a hollow organ like the intestines or stomach.

Sphincter A ring of muscle that surrounds an opening or tube in the body and helps to close it on contracting. E.g., Anal sphincter.

Spotting Any uterine or vaginal bleeding that occurs outside the menstrual period.

Stem cell Cells present in the Bone Marrow which can grow into different types of cells like red cells, white cells, platelets etc. A stem cell is an immature cell which can differentiate into any type of cell in the body. E.g., Nerve cells, Muscle cells, Bone cells etc.

Stools Feces : Poop : Excrement.

Stricture A narrowing or constriction of the cavity of a hollow organ or tube. E.g., Urethra, Esophagus, Ureter.

Suppository A solid compound like glycerin or cocoa butter which contains medication which is released when the compound melts inside the body. Inserted into the Rectum, Vagina or Urethra.

Swab A wad of absorbent material like cotton, wound to the end of a small stick used to take samples from wounds or from pus for laboratory examination. They are also used to apply medicines to areas.

Tartar A hard, whitish, calcified deposit that forms on teeth and gums.

Thermoregulation The mechanism by which the body maintains its internal temperature by self-regulation irrespective of the external temperature.

Thrombocyte Platelets : Tiny disc shaped cells seen in blood.

Thrombocytopenia A condition where the platelet count in blood is too low.

Tinea captitis Ringworm of the scalp caused by fungal infection.
Tinea corporis Ringworm of the body.
Tinea manuum Fungal infection of the hands and palms.

Tinea pedis Athlete's Foot : Fungal infection occurring between the toes.

Tinea unguium Fungal infection of the nails.

Transvaginal Ultrasound An ultrasound scan where an instrument is inserted into the vagina to examine the uterus, cervix , ovaries, Fallopian tubes, and bladder.

Ulcer An open sore on the external or internal surface of the body caused by a break in the skin or mucous membrane.

Ultrasound scan An imaging procedure using High Frequency Sound waves (Ultra Sound) to image the organs of the body.

Urologist A doctor specialized in the diagnosis and treatment of the disorders of the Urinary system.

Uterus Womb : The pear-shaped hollow organ in the pelvis on women where the fertilized egg grows into a full blown baby.

Vertigo A sensation of spinning or whirling with loss of balance.

Vesicle A small fluid filled swelling on the skin : Blister.

Villi (Sing: Villus) Small, slender, finger-like projections in the inner lining of the small intestines.

Visual Acuity Clarity or sharpness of vision to see things clearly.

Vitreous A gel like fluid that fills the inside of the eye : Vitreous means "glass-like"

Vulva The outer part of the female genitals.
Vulvovaginitis Inflammation of the vulva and vagina due to infection.
W.H.O. World Health Organization.

Xerosis Abnormal dryness of part of a body or tissue. E.g., Skin, Conjunctiva, Oral cavity.

Xerostomia Dryness of mouth due to inadequate saliva production.

ACKNOWLEDGEMENTS

I sincerely thank Drs. Abhay Martin and Dr. Rajmohan who provided references for the chapters on Skin Disorders and Psychiatric disorders respectively.

I place on record my sincere thanks to Prof. M.R. Rajagopal, Chairman, Pallium India for his valuable advice and inputs regarding the latest update on Advanced Medical Directive in India. Prof. R. Krishnan helped me in getting these details promptly. My thanks are due to him.

My family has always stood by me and put up with my foibles while writing this book. I gracefully acknowledge their role .

The cover for the book was designed by Lolitha of Ravendesigns. I thank her for the beautiful and eye-catching design.

I gratefully acknowledge the advice from Mr. Vikram Khaitan, who is an active member of the author community and has been kind enough to suggest the catchy title for this book.

Above all, I must place on record my sincere thanks to Mr. Som Bathla, my mentor in this author journey and all the enthusiastic members of the Author-Helping-Author (AHA) community who have always given me constructive suggestions and encouragement at various stages of my writing and publishing.

ABOUT THE AUTHOR

The author is a practicing Cardiologist. In this book he writes about the *Problems of the Elderly* individuals. This is written in two parts, this being Part 2 of the book. In a simple, non-medical language, he deals with the medical problems facing the elderly population.

He has written two previous books of Short Stories with morals, mainly for children named **'Tell Me A Story, Grandpa'** and **'Grandpa, Tell Me More Stories.'** His third book **'In Search of a Bridegroom'** is an Autobiographical fiction based on his personal experiences.

His book titled, **"How to Face the Health Challenges While Growing Old"** is the Part 1 of the series *'Problems of the Elderly'* and was published three months ago. It deals with some of the diseases and problems of Old Age. This book is a sequel to the first book describing more body systems and their disorders.

Other books by the Author

Tell Me A Story, Grandpa

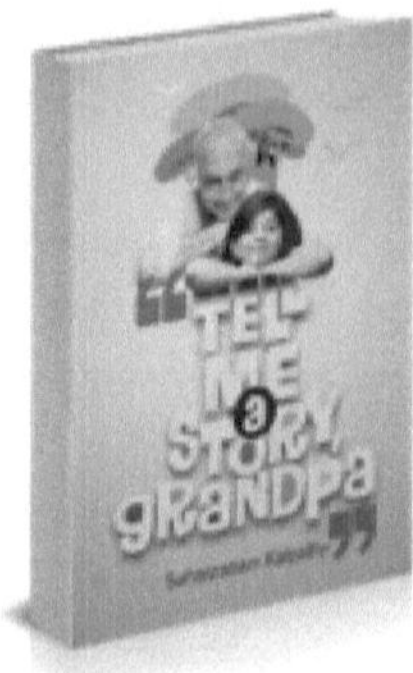

This is the first book written by the author in his 'Grandpa Series'.

Grandpa tirelessly regales children with forty stories from all around. Every story carries a moral at the end for the children to ruminate upon. These stories can keep your children engaged and fascinated during their free time.

"There is a good reason for everything that happens", says Grandpa, "Like the story of the ship-wrecked sailor" and the children immediately pounce upon grandpa to tell them the story of the Ship-wrecked Sailor.

"Don't interfere with your dad while he is painting the patio, your advice is not needed," says Grandpa, "Like the King's Sculptor who was advised by too many people".

There are stories which inculcate Benevolence (The Three Good Deeds), Dedication (Akbar and Tansen) Humility (The Humble Millionaire), Devotion to God (God's Grace), and stories Just for Laughs (The Cure, Oh! Doctor)

And many more such stories in the backdrop of everyday occurrence in the families as a prelude which takes you to the height of imagination and morality.

Other books by the Author
Grandpa, Tell Me More Stories

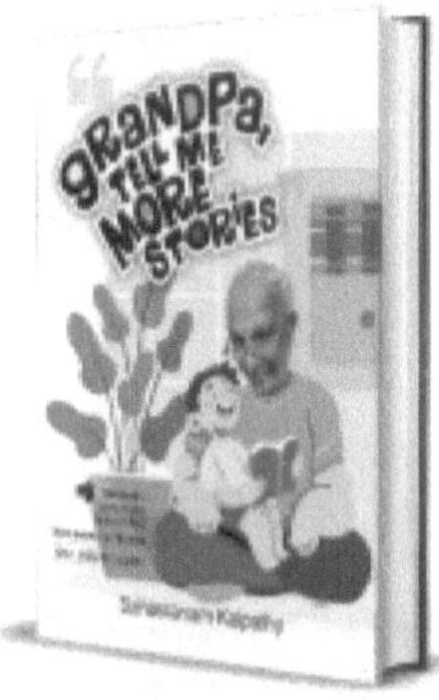

This is a collection of forty short stories for children. It is a continuation of the previous book where Grandpa regales his granddaughters with more moral-packed stories. The stories are derived from various sources and endeavour to instil values of truth, justice, and honesty in children.

Do you find that your children are bored? Read them these short stories with Morals, Educational and Entertaining. Both Fiction and Mythology stories are presented. Humorous stories and thought-provoking ones keep the children engaged and enthralled. They make ideal bedtime stories for kids.

Both books promise to keep your children entertained during their holidays. The books form an ideal gift to be given to children on their birthdays.

The book is a must read by every child and should be the part of every school library.

Other books by the Author
In Search Of A Bridegroom

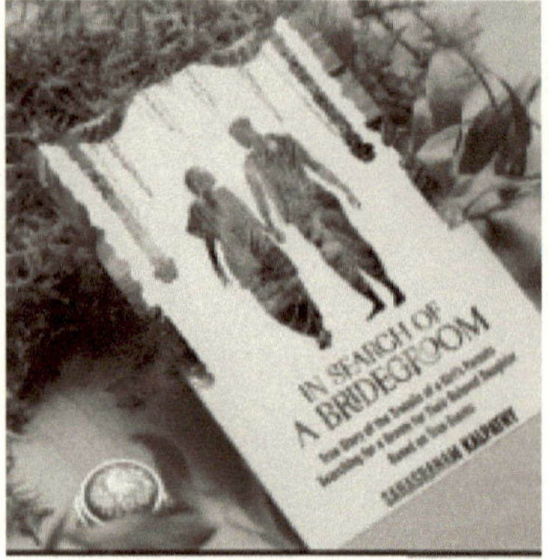

This is the third book by the author and describes the problems faced by a parent when he begins searching for an appropriate bridegroom for his daughter.

This is the story of every parent in India and the author portrays the woes of a concerned parent in this 'Autobiographical fiction'.

Once a daughter reaches a marriageable age, it is the duty of the parents to find a suitable bridegroom for her. This is the tradition in Hindu culture. Certain sects of Hindus have rigid rules regarding marriage and choice of a bridegroom. The author, himself a Tamil Brahmin, thought-provokingly chronicles the not-so-pleasant experiences encountered while searching for a suitable boy for his daughter.

The events described in this book are true and takes the readers through a real time accounts of the events as they unfolded revealing the attitudes and chicanery of some individuals.

Other books by the Author
How to Face the Health Challenges While Growing Old

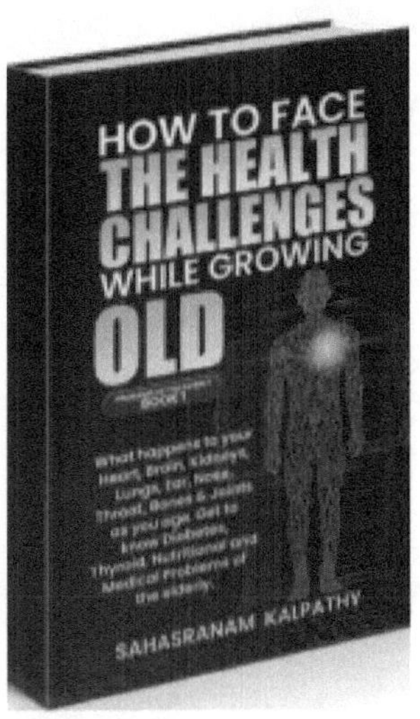

Growing old in an inevitable part of life. Old age brings many changes in the human body. One should be aware of these changes to grow old gracefully. This is the Book 1 of the series "Problems of the Elderly".

Diseases of the Heart, Brain, Lungs, and Kidneys are common when one grows old. So are diseases of the Thyroid gland, Ear, Nose, Throat, Bones and Joints.

Diabetes and Nutritional Diseases of Old Age need special attention. All these have been comprehensively discussed in the book.

The Symptoms, Diagnosis and the Treatment of these diseases have been elaborated in simple English avoiding the medical terminology as far as possible.

The Precautions to be taken and the Preventive measures needed are explained explicitly.

To aid the reader, a Glossary is included at the end of the book explaining some of the terms used in the book.

Illustrative Diagrams are used wherever possible to make the understanding of the structure of the organs and systems simple.

The Book 1 is a companion to the present book and together they form a series on *Problems of the Elderly*.